Understanding Physician–Pharmaceutical Industry Interactions

Physician–pharmaceutical industry interactions continue to generate heated debate in academic and public domains, both in the United States and abroad. Despite this, recent research suggests that physicians and physicians-in-training remain ignorant of the core issues and are ill-prepared to understand pharmaceutical industry promotion. Furthermore, few medical curricula cover this issue, despite warnings of the imperative need to address this gap in the education of tomorrow's physicians. There is a vast medical literature on this topic, but no single, concise resource. This book aims to fill that gap by providing a resource that explains the essential elements of this subject. The text makes the reader more aware of the key ethical issues and allows the reader to be a more savvy interpreter of industry promotion, have a heightened awareness of the public and medical legal consequences of some physician–pharmaceutical industry interactions and be better equipped to handle real-life encounters with industry.

Shaili Jain, MD, attended Liverpool Medical School in England and completed her postgraduate training in the United States. She currently works as a General Adult Psychiatrist with Aurora Behavioral Health Services and is also Clinical Assistant Professor of Psychiatry at the Medical College of Wisconsin in Milwaukee.

Understanding Physician–Pharmaceutical Industry Interactions

Shaili Jain, MD

General Adult Psychiatrist
Aurora Behavioral Health Services
Milwaukee, Wisconsin

Clinical Assistant Professor of Psychiatry
Medical College of Wisconsin
Milwaukee, Wisconsin

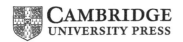

CAMBRIDGE
UNIVERSITY PRESS

CAMBRIDGE
UNIVERSITY PRESS

University Printing House, Cambridge CB2 8BS, United Kingdom

One Liberty Plaza, 20th Floor, New York, NY 10006, USA

477 Williamstown Road, Port Melbourne, VIC 3207, Australia

314-321, 3rd Floor, Plot 3, Splendor Forum, Jasola District Centre, New Delhi - 110025, India

79 Anson Road, #06-04/06, Singapore 079906

Cambridge University Press is part of the University of Cambridge.

It furthers the University's mission by disseminating knowledge in the pursuit of education, learning and research at the highest international levels of excellence.

www.cambridge.org
Information on this title: www.cambridge.org/9780521688666

First published 2007

A catalogue record for this publication is available from the British Library

Library of Congress Cataloging in Publication data
Jain, Shaili, 1974–
Understanding physician–pharmaceutical industry interaction / Shaili Jain.
  p. ; cm.
Includes index.
ISBN 978-0-521-86864-8 (hardback) – ISBN 978-0-521-68866-6 (pbk.)
  1. Physicians – Professional ethics.   2. Pharmaceutical industry – Moral and
ethical aspects.   3. Drugs – Marketing.   4. Advertising – Drugs.   I. Title.
[DNLM: 1. Physicians – ethics.   2. Advertising.   3. Drug Industry – ethics.
4. Gift Giving – ethics. W 62 J25U 2007]   I. Title.
R727.5.J35   2007
174.2′951 – dc22   2006037016

ISBN 978-0-521-86864-8 Hardback
ISBN 978-0-521-68866-6 Paperback

....

Contents

Contents

Acknowledgments

―――――――――――――――――

The author wishes to express deep appreciation to Carlyle H. Chan, MD; Kidar Nath Jain; Joseph Layde, MD, JD; Jon Lehrmann, MD and Anthony Meyer, MD, for their careful review of various parts of this manuscript and very helpful suggestions in preparation of this work.

Foreword

Understanding Physician–Pharmaceutical Industry Interactions is a long-overdue book summarizing deliberations that have spanned many years. I am a PGY (postgraduate year) 51; Dr. Shaili Jain is a PGY 8. Although two generations apart, we are in complete agreement with the need for coalesced thinking about the conflicts of self-interest in the relationship between the pharmaceutical industry and the profession of medicine. Dr. Jain is to be complimented for undertaking this subject that has undoubtedly caused her consternation as a young physician.

This topic is very important for all health professionals who prescribe medicines or medical devices. Health care now consumes $2 trillion annually and is approaching 17% of the gross national product. And, as the costs continue to escalate, individuals, families, industry, and businesses and municipal, county, state and federal governments falter economically. Prescribing medical professionals, who are responsible for at least 75% of the annual cost of health care, unfortunately are often unaware of the cost of the drugs, tests, services and supplies they prescribe. The patients, except for their co-payments, are uninterested because of the confusion and complexities of billing, and, after all, a third party is responsible for payment. To curtail the rising cost of health care, everyone *must* become cost conscious. No other service or product is purchased so blindly.

Business ethics are different from medical ethics. In the business climate it is common for industry to reward and entice their vendors in order to stimulate sales. The pharmaceutical industry has a similar culture, and at its interface and overlap with the medical profession, what the pharmaceutical industry formally considers normal business behavior, the medical profession considers unethical. It is estimated that the pharmaceutical industry spends $14 billion per annum in marketing. According to statistics, there is one pharmaceutical representative for every nine physicians. It is a huge force. This, coupled with direct-to-consumer advertising, in which the bottom line is always "ask your doctor if this medicine is good for you," places the prescriber under increasing pressure. Medical ethics prompt physicians to consider that if current promotional activities such as inviting physicians to expensive dinners, parties, trips, entertainment and even office lunches as well as direct-to-consumer advertising were eliminated, the money saved could be used to lower the cost of drugs to the benefit of our patients. *Understanding Physician–Pharmaceutical Industry Interactions* outlines current thinking and guidelines for accomplishing that goal.

When I studied pharmacology in medical school, it was stressed that physicians should familiarize themselves with selected drugs, learn to understand them well and prescribe as few medicines as expeditiously as possible. Based on experience, we were taught to continue to use those medicines that were therapeutically effective, had a wide margin of safety and were least expensive among their class. These principles hold true today.

The American Medical Association was founded in 1847 for the purpose of developing a code of medical ethics to promote professionalism. Today the AMA's Council on Ethical and Judicial Affairs (CEJA) is responsible for the AMA's *Code of Medical Ethics*, a volume updated and published biannually. The current Code includes approximately 180 Opinions (www.ama-assn.org/go/ceja). All Opinions relate to the nine time-honored Principles of Medical Ethics. Opinion 8.061, entitled "Gifts to Physicians from Industry" and adopted by the AMA's House of Delegates in 1990, offers guidelines regarding gifts from the pharmaceutical industry to physicians. Gifts should not be of substantial value, should relate to the physician's work, should be educational and scholarly and should not involve direct or indirect exchange of currency.

In 1999, a task force entitled the Working Group for Communication of Ethical Guidelines on Gifts to Physicians from Industry was convened. The following organizations were represented: Accreditation Council for Continuing Medical Education; Adva Med, Inc.; Alliance for Continuing Medical Education; American Academy of Family Practice; American Academy of Pediatrics; American College of Obstetricians and Gynecologists; American College of Physicians; American College of Surgeons; American Medical Association; American Medical Association Industry Roundtable Steering Committee; American Osteopathic Association; American Psychiatric Association; American Society of Anesthesiology; AstraZeneca International; Bayer Corporation; Coalition for Healthcare Communication; Council of Medical Specialty Societies; Eli Lilly and Company; GlaxoSmithKline; Merck & Company, Inc.; National Medical Association; Pfizer; Inc.; Pharmaceutical Research and Manufacturers of America; Pharmacia Corporation; Physicians World/Thompson Healthcare; Procter & Gamble Pharmaceuticals; Society for Academic Continuing Medical Education; United States Department of Veterans Affairs and Wyeth-Ayerst Laboratories. After review and meeting for approximately three years, it was agreed and promulgated that CEJA Opinion 8.061 entitled "Gifts to Physicians from Industry" was an acceptable guideline to which all parties would adhere.

In my library I have a copy of William Osler's volume *Aequanimitas with Other Addresses*, which was a gift to all medical school graduates in 1932 from Eli Lilly and Company and includes a letter inscribed by Mr. Eli Lilly, the company president, that reads as follows:

May 1932

Dear Doctor,

Together with congratulations on your attainment of a medical degree, this volume of addresses by Sir William Osler, who adorned your profession in the United States for so many years, is cordially presented.

As the addresses by this master mind of modern medicine are read, may you catch his vision of the almost boundless possibilities of your profession.

May you share with him his "relish of knowledge" and his absorbing love and passionate search for truth.

Above all, may there come to you an inspiration which will enable you to live a rich, a happy and an abundant life.

Sincerely yours,

Eli Lilly and Company
Eli Lilly
President

I consider a gift of this nature to be a thoughtful expression. It is an inexpensive gift, but a valuable and useful reference for a physician's lifetime and beyond.

The achievements in medicine during the 20th century were spectacular. Life expectancy in the United States has nearly doubled in 100 years. In the past 50 years, we have seen the conquest of poliomyelitis and the transplantation of organs, among so many other achievements. Society benefits from brilliant minds in basic science, medicine and pharmacology working collaboratively. It is said of the late Dr. Maurice R. Hilleman that he saved many lives with the development of 40 vaccines that have eliminated or significantly reduced the occurrence of many communicable diseases. Dr. Hilleman, who had a PhD degree, worked most of his professional life for Merck & Co.

In order to continue to advance along the road of discovery, the pharmaceutical industry and the medical profession must work in synergy. The relationship must be completely devoid of conflict of self-interest and greed. And the relationship between the prescriber of medicines and the pharmaceutical manufacturers (and their representatives) must not be self-serving for either. It is all about the patient and the betterment of society.

I think every young physician should have the opportunity to tour a pharmaceutical manufacturing company and marvel at and better appreciate the elaborateness and complexities of the drug production process. Bridging the chasm within the framework of science, ethics, service and professionalism will encourage mutual appreciation and respect.

This book, written by a young psychiatrist, brings it all into focus.

It should serve to strengthen the importance of collaboration within the boundaries of ethics and professionalism. Upholding ethics and professionalism will, and should, solidify the matrix of the healing occupations.

Leonard J. Morse, MD
Commissioner of Public Health, City of Worcester,
Massachusetts, USA

Professor of Clinical Medicine,
Family Medicine and Community Health,
University of Massachusetts Medical School.

Past member and Chair, Council on Ethical and Judicial Affairs,
American Medical Association
September 8, 2006

Introduction

Why Write a Book about Physician– Pharmaceutical Industry Interactions (PPIIs)?[1]

These interactions have consequences for patients, doctors and the larger society [1]. These interactions are frequent and involve more than just a face-to-face visit with a pharmaceutical company representative (PCR). Moynihan referred to these interactions as "entanglements," and examples are listed in Figure 0.1. The budgets of the pharmaceutical industry (PI)[2] support many of the PPIIs, such as paying PCR salaries, providing free gifts for physicians and subsidizing funding for continuing medical education (CME). The marketing expenditure of the U.S. drug industry reached $15.7 billion in 2000 [2] with nearly one PCR and almost $100,000 for every eleven practicing physicians in the United States [3]. With the number of new medications coming onto the market only increasing, physicians are finding it hard to keep up to date, and many find that utilizing

---

[1] This term was first used in the literature by Watkins RS, Kimberly J. Acad Med 2004; 79:432–7

[2] The term *pharmaceutical industry* is interchangeable with *pharmaceutical equipment manufacturers*.

industry-supplied sources of information can be a convenient and easy way of staying current in their daily practice. As government funds diminish in academic settings and industry investment increases, this subject is likely to remain an important issue for the medical profession to study and understand [2].

Who Should Read This Book?

This book should be read by any physician or medical trainee who has engaged in any of the interactions outlined in Figure 0.1, as well

---

Forms of Entanglement

☐ Face-to-face visits from drug company representatives
☐ Acceptance of direct gifts of equipment, travel or accommodation
☐ Acceptance of indirect gifts, through sponsorship of software or travel
☐ Attendance at sponsored dinners and social or recreational events
☐ Attendance at sponsored educational events, continuing medical education, workshops or seminars
☐ Attendance at sponsored scientific conferences
☐ Ownership of stock or equity holdings
☐ Conducting sponsored research
☐ Company funding for medical schools, academic chairs, or lecture halls
☐ Membership in sponsored professional societies and associations
☐ Advising a sponsored disease foundation or patients' group
☐ Involvement with or use of sponsored clinical guidelines
☐ Undertaking paid consultancy work for companies
☐ Membership of company advisory boards of "thought leaders" or "speakers' bureaus"
☐ Authoring "ghostwritten" scientific articles
☐ Reading medical journals that rely on drug company advertising, company-purchased reprints and sponsored supplements

---

Figure 0.1
Table taken from "Who pays for the pizza?" Redefining the relationships between doctors and drug companies 1: Entanglement BMJ 2003; 326:31. Reprinted with the permission of BMJ Publishing Company.

as by other health care professionals such as nurses, nurse prescribers, physician assistants and pharmacists who have such interactions with the PI and a significant influence on patient perceptions of prescription medications.

Why Should I Read This Book?

PPIIs on an individual basis are frequent; they begin in medical school and persist through a physician's career.

Outside of one-on-one interactions, the relationship of industry with the medical establishment is extensive: funding of research trials, subsidizing CME and advertisements in major medical journals.

There is considerable empirical data proving that physician judgment and prescribing is compromised and negatively influenced if these physicians are recipients of gifts from the pharmaceutical industry.

This data as well as increasing public scrutiny of these interactions has prompted many medical societies and professional organizations to offer position statements and policies on these issues.

Despite all this, most physicians at various levels of training remain unaware of the data or the policies and uninformed on how to conduct ethical relationships with the PI and PCRs.

The debate about PPIIs is not only a professional debate but also a public one, with much media scrutiny and legal consequences of problematic PPIIs.

This book aims to heighten the reader's awareness about PPIIs, the nature of these interactions and their advantages and disadvantages in a variety of medical settings. The hope is that this will increase the reader's "promotional literacy": that it will fine-tune the reader's ability to separate true science from sophisticated promotion and thus better serve our patients.

Clinical vignettes revolving around four fictional characters support the material in these chapters. Brenda Balant is a PCR for the company Brown Pharmaceuticals, promoting the new antihypertensive drug Lowpress. Jack Jones is a senior internal medicine resident with aspirations to become a cardiologist. Bob Brunswick is a PCR for the company MedCorp and is promoting the new antidepressant Vivre. Jane Jensan is a family practice resident with a special interest in psychiatry.

References

1. Blumenthal D. Doctors and drug companies. N Engl J Med 2004; 351(18):1885–90

2. Wazana A, Primeau F. Ethical considerations in the relationship between physicians and the pharmaceutical industry. Psychiatr Clin North Am 2002; 25(3):647–63, viii

3. Zuger A. Fever pitch: Getting doctors to prescribe is big business. The New York Times. Jan 11, 1999. Late Edition, Section A, Page 1, Column 4

1 Gifts from the Pharmaceutical Industry to Physicians

Do They Influence Your Prescribing?

Brenda is in a good mood. She has been trying to get an invitation to sponsor breakfast at the internal medicine grand rounds for several weeks and just got a phone call from the grand rounds coordinator, Gloria, confirming an opening for the following week. Brenda is very keen to meet the residents, especially the new PGY 1 class. Experience has taught her that targeting younger physicians who are not set in their prescribing ways pays off. Furthermore, once they start prescribing her medication they tend to stay loyal to the brand. She wants to talk to them about Lowpress, her new medication for the treatment of hypertension. She also enjoys working with residents, as she finds it easy to socialize and chat with them: many of them are similar to her in age and share common interests with her. Hosting breakfast at grand rounds will give her good exposure to the residents. She already knows the caterer she will use; she has overheard the residents raving about the pastries there. Experience has also taught her that well-satisfied stomachs make for better listeners!

In 2000, pharmaceutical companies spent $15.7 billion promoting their products, with 84% directed toward medical promotions via detailing, drug samples and journal ads [1]. Promotional dollars spent on "gifts" for physicians are ubiquitous in medical environments, with one study showing that 97% of residents carried at least one item with a pharmaceutical company logo on it [2]. Across cultures and over time, it has been observed that gift exchange stimulates social advancement by creating networks. Giving a gift creates a social contract and imposes a reciprocal obligation, even if the gift is unwanted and the giver is distrusted or disliked [3]. Reciprocation is so highly valued a social norm that those who do not reciprocate are often regarded with disgust and assigned negative labels [4]. In addition, the gift givers, in this case pharmaceutical company representatives (PCRs), are usually bright, young and personable. This makes it hard not to like them, and industry's public relations experts know the importance of these personal contacts [5].

Types of Gifts

Small gifts such as pens, message pads, and office clocks are accepted by nearly all physicians [4]. Individual physicians may receive these items, which bear the company or product name, and also more expensive items such as medical books and medical equipment [6]. Gifts such as pens and notepads are called "reminder items"; they play an important role in opening doors and promoting friendlier, more cooperative relationships between the pharmaceutical company representative and physician [4].

The pharmaceutical industry (PI) often provides free meals and refreshments at medical conferences, schools and hospitals. Conference organizers often solicit subsidies in order to increase attendance at events. Food, flattery and friendship are all powerful tools of persuasion, particularly when combined. The act of dining helps to foster cozier working relationships that might help break down professional barriers between physicians and sales representatives [4].

Industry-supplied free medication samples for medical clinics as well as for the personal use of physicians and their family members are another example of gifts. (See Chapter 9.)

The PI may support hospital conferences by paying honoraria and travel expenses for speakers. These subsidies enable schools or hospitals to invite nationally prominent speakers [6]. Gifts such as textbooks that support educational advancement of physicians can be seen as beneficial to patient care. Reduced availability of government funds for education has led to substantial increases in commercial support for educational activities, and the resultant conflict between product promotion and "education" has been highlighted in the literature by leading academics [7, 8].

There are many arguments supporting gift giving from industry to physicians. The act promotes goodwill between physicians and the pharmaceutical industry, and the relationship between physicians and industry can result in impressive medical advances [9]. On an educational front, it has been hypothesized that without free meals many potential attendees would not be present at continuing medical education events and would remain ignorant of new advances [10]. Industry spokesmen have argued that sales representatives can be viewed as performing a valuable function that promotes better patient care, at a time when doctors are bombarded daily with new information and are finding it difficult to keep up to date [11]. In the past, it was felt that "arguments presented against the moral permissibility of these relationships (between pharmaceutical industry representatives and physicians) were wanting and poorly formulated" [12]. Furthermore, there is no evidence that physicians knowingly or intentionally compromise their patients' care as a result of gifts from the industry; the vast majority of physicians are able to resist this temptation and make decisions solely based on the best medical interest of their patients [10, 11]. According to PhRMA (Pharmaceutical Research and Manufacturers of America), the exchange of gifts is balanced because they are compensation for the time physicians spend becoming educated about products.

Arguments against gift giving are that these relations create opportunities for bias and can result in unfavorable public perceptions, overconsumption and misuse of public money. Also, "the profession (medical) needs to be suspicious of pure merchandising since we not only enjoy patients' confidence but the confidence of the entire society" [10]. Furthermore, the physician's role is seen as fiduciary; that is, "a physician holds the trust and confidence of the patient and is empowered to act in the patient's best interest." If physicians' prescribing practices are influenced by pharmaceutical company incentives rather than by objective medical evidence, then the physician is not solely acting in the patient's best interest [13]. In 2000 Wazana conducted a landmark analysis of more than 20 studies, which concluded that free gifts affect physicians' prescribing behavior typically in a negative way: for example, erroneous knowledge regarding the medication, rapid prescription of a new drug, formulary requests for newer medications that rarely hold an advantage over existing ones, and nonrational prescribing [14]. There remains an additional argument that even if there is no actual effect on a physician's prescribing behavior, there might be a public impression of impropriety of this activity [10]. In counterpoint to the argument that gifts are given in exchange for physicians' time, this exchange can also be seen as a negative one because the practice is inherently profit motivated, and profit potential significantly exceeds the value of the gift [4].

> Jack is feeling stressed. He has just finished a night on call. It was his first night as senior resident leading the medical team. The night had been hectic with a steady stream of admissions from the ER. Jack feels slightly anxious about rounds. He is keen to impress the attending, who is an eminent cardiologist with a reputation for impeccably high expectations for the trainees who work for him. Jack's intern, although trying hard, was slow and Jack had to stay up with him so they could get through the work. To add to Jack's stress, his wife had been paging him intermittently to give him updates on the well-being of their two-year-old son who is sick with an ear infection. As he heads to grand rounds, he hopes a drug rep will be hosting breakfast. He needs a pickup to get him through the rest of the morning and did not fancy an additional trip to the drab hospital

cafeteria. He is glad to find his favorite pastries being served and also happy to see Brenda. She is always cheerful and pleasant and often asks about his wife and children. She is handing out literature on a new hypertensive medication. Jack picks up a selection of delicious pastries and a cup of coffee and heads over to talk with Brenda about the new medicine...maybe he will be able to impress the team on rounds with this up-to-date information.

Summary

☐ Gift giving from the pharmaceutical industry to physicians is a frequent occurrence in medical environments.
☐ The exchanges of such gifts occur frequently in medical settings.
☐ Values of the gifts vary from small items (e.g., pens) to larger gifts (e.g., subsidizing medical conferences).
☐ There is empirical data proving that such gifts influence physician prescribing in negative ways.

References

1. Rosenthal MB, Berndt ER, Donohue JM, Frank RG, Epstein AM. Promotion of prescription drugs to consumers. N Engl J Med 2002; 346(7): 498–505

2. Sigworth SK, Nettleman MD, Cohen GM. Pharmaceutical branding of resident physicians. JAMA 2001; 286(9):1024–5

3. Katz D, Mansfield P, Goodman R, Tiefer L, Merz J. Psychological aspects of gifts from drug companies. JAMA 2003; 290(18):2404–5

4. Katz D, Caplan AL, Merz JF. All gifts large and small. Am J Bioethics 2003; 3(3):39–46

5. Rhodes R, Capozzi JD. The invisible influence of industry inducements. Am J Bioethics 2003; 3(3):65–7

6. Lo B. *Resolving Ethical Dilemmas: A Guide for Clinicians*. Williams & Wilkins, Baltimore, 1995

7. Relman AS. Separating continuing medical education from pharmaceutical marketing. JAMA 2001; 285(15):2009–12

8. Stahl S. It takes two to entangle: Separating medical education from pharmaceutical promotion. Psychopharmacology Educational Update. 2005 (March):1, 6

9. Goodwin FK. Safe and effective drugs have improved the lives of millions. Psychol Today 1999; 32(5):40–2

10. Desmet C. Pharmaceuticals firms' generosity and physicians: Legal aspects in Belgium. Med Law 2003; 22(3):473–87

11. Spilker B. The benefits and risks of a packet of M&M's. Health Aff 2002; 21(2):243–4

12. Peppin JF. Pharmaceutical sales representatives and physicians: Ethical considerations of a relationship. J Med Philos 1996; 21(1):83–99

13. Williams SC. Food for thought. Why physicians should reconsider gifts from pharmaceutical companies. Curr Surg 2003; 60(2):152–3

14. Wazana A. Physicians and the pharmaceutical industry: Is a gift ever just a gift? JAMA 2000; 283(3):373–80

2 Ethical Considerations of Receiving Gifts from the Pharmaceutical Industry

Brenda had had a busy afternoon. Her company had provided funds for two internal medicine residents to attend a national cardiology conference in New York. Even though nominations of the residents and payment for the event were coordinated through the department, Brenda was keen to spend some time with the chosen residents at the conference. She had successfully contacted one of them, Jack, and invited him and his colleague to dinner the evening before the conference. Brenda knew from her chats with Gloria, the residency coordinator, that Jack was a highly valued resident with aspirations to be a cardiologist. She was keen to talk to him more about the new antihypertensive medication Lowpress. The dinner would be an ideal opportunity to do this, so Brenda set about booking a table at one of the finest restaurants in New York.

Prescribing medication is not a simple technical action; it is a complex social interaction with many levels of meaning. Ethical medication giving requires an awareness of the importance and the inevitability of these many layers of meaning and their effects [1]. Physicians who receive free gifts from the pharmaceutical industry need to be aware of the ethical issues that are raised and their possible effects on the action of prescribing.

Conflict of Interest

Physicians have an ethical duty to serve the interests of their patients and to avoid potential conflicts that might divert them from that commitment [2]. For the sake of argument, even if gifts did not influence physicians, public trust in the medical profession might be compromised [3]. This is echoed in the results of a patient survey showing that a substantial majority believed that gifts influence physician prescribing at least sometimes [4]. This issue has been addressed in the ethical policy of the American Medical Association concerning gifts to physicians from industry, which emphasizes that any gifts accepted by individual physicians should primarily entail a benefit to patients. This emphasizes physicians' professional obligation to place patients' interests above their own [5].

Impairment of Objectivity

Social science research shows that even when individuals try to be objective, their judgments are subject to an unconscious and unintentional self-serving bias. Furthermore, individuals are generally unaware of the bias, so they do not make efforts to correct for it or to avoid conflicts of interest in the first place [6]. Patients surveyed tended to find gifts less appropriate and more influential than did their physicians [7]. The best predictor of a patient feeling gifts were inappropriate was the belief that those gifts might influence prescribing. Seventy percent of patients in another study believed gifts sometimes or frequently influence prescribing [4]. Furthermore, many physicians do not appreciate how commercial information significantly influences their patient care decisions [3]. Despite much data to show the influence of industry on physician belief and behaviors, the majority of physicians believe that they are not influenced by drug companies. In addition, there is evidence we can see the resultant bias in our colleagues but not ourselves [8].

Jack had just arrived at his hotel in New York. He was really looking forward to the conference as well as a chance to have a mini break. He had been very pleased that his program director had nominated him and his close buddy Raj for the trip. He never could have afforded to attend if Brown Pharmaceuticals had not covered the expenses, and he was truly grateful for the opportunity. There was a voice mail from Brenda on his hotel phone giving him the details of the restaurant where they would be meeting for dinner. An hour later Jack, Raj and Brenda were having cocktails in an elegant New York restaurant. This feels really good, Jack thought to himself. He could not remember the last time he had been in a place like this. Busy nights on call and a hectic home life with twin boy toddlers did not often accommodate such evenings out. He expressed his gratitude, again, to Brenda. Over dessert and coffee Brenda talked about Low-press, the company's latest antihypertensive medication. Jack was impressed with her presentation of studies showing that the medication had less troublesome side effects than some of the other medications on the market. He was not exactly sure how this translated clinically but nonetheless was keen to give it a try.

Cost of Health Care

A third of patients surveyed and 64% of respondents in another study believed that gifts to physicians from the pharmaceutical industry (PI) increase the cost of medications [3, 4, 7]. Consumer advocates believe that the public needs to know about gifts from the drug companies to physicians. A suggested rule of thumb is, "What would your patients or the public think if they knew you had accepted such gifts?"[3]. What is the purpose of the industry offer? What would I think if my own doctor or colleagues accepted this offer?[9].

Summary

☐ Physicians who receive free gifts from the pharmaceutical industry must consider the ethical dilemmas posed by this practice.

☐ These dilemmas are conflict of interest, impairment of objectivity and the impact of these free gifts on the cost of health care.

☐ Physicians do not always see the resultant bias in their prescribing even though social science research and other empirical data have proven it does exist.

☐ Patients frequently feel that gifts from the pharmaceutical industry influence physician prescribing and contribute to rising health care costs.

References

1. Jonsen AR. Ethics of drug giving and drug taking. Drug Issues 1988; 18(2):195–200

2. Brody H. The company we keep: Why physicians should refuse to see pharmaceutical representatives. Ann Fam Med 2005; 3(1):82–5

3. Lo B. *Resolving Ethical Dilemmas: A Guide for Clinicians.* Williams & Wilkins, Baltimore, 1995

4. Blake RL, Early EK. Patients' attitudes about gifts to physicians from pharmaceutical companies. J Am Board Fam Pract 1995; 8(6):457–64

5. Goldrich MS. Psychological aspects of gifts from drug companies. JAMA 2003; 290(18):2405

6. Dana J, Loewenstein G. A social science perspective on gifts to physicians from industry. JAMA; 290(2):252–5

7. Gibbons RV, Landry FJ, Blouch DL, Jones DL, Williams FK, Lucey CR, Kroenke K. A comparison of physicians' and patients' attitudes toward pharmaceutical industry gifts. J Gen Intern Med 1998; 13(3): 151–4

8. Steinman MA, Shilipak MG, McPhee SJ. Of principles and pens: Attitudes and practices of medicine housestaff toward pharmaceutical industry promotions. Am J Med 2001; 110(7):551–7

9. Gudmundsson S. Doctors and drug companies: The beauty and the beast. Acta Ophthalmol Scand 2005; 83:407–8

3

One on One

An Analysis of the Physician–

Pharmaceutical Company

Representative (PCR) Detailing

Interaction

The Nature of Detailing

Historically, the method of promotion that has proven most effective for the pharmaceutical industry is the process of detailing, in which PCRs visit physician offices to discuss the availability and suitability of products [1]. PCRs are the link between the company and the physician. They contact an average of 8–10 medical offices in a day with the goal of influencing physicians to prescribe their company's brands [2]. In recent years, sales representative presence has apparently increased significantly [3], with 83% of physicians in one study acknowledging visits from PCRs regardless of physician age, gender and specialty [4].

In 1998 the pharmaceutical industry (PI) spent $12.724 billion on promotion in the United States, with $3.537 billion on office promotion [5]. Constant interactions build a stock of goodwill between a PCR and the physician, and this changes physician prescription behavior in a "positive" way (i.e., favorable to the company) [6].

The importance of an actual relationship between PCR and physician has been highlighted in marketing journals. "Loyalty to a PCR who has become a friend to the physician may prove stronger than loyalty to the brand" [7]. This philosophy may help to explain why, historically, there has been much emphasis placed on the choice of proper personnel to act as emissaries for the company: for example, "have a good appearance, pleasing personality, moderate habits, good health and physical fitness" [3, 8].

Services provided by PCRs include providing free product samples, detailing new products, inviting physicians to promotional dinners, sponsoring office lunches and providing product studies or research findings [2, 3]. In one study, provision of free samples was considered to be the single most important service provided by PCRs [2]. (For more details, please refer to Chapter 9.)

Physician Responses to Detailing

There is ample evidence that physicians are influenced by sales presentations and associated kindnesses such as free gifts and food. This influence can lead to bad prescribing habits [9]. Despite these data, detailing flourishes, as it provides an inexpensive and convenient source of information. Physicians surveyed regarded detailing as more influential on prescribing than seminars, conferences, advertisements in journals or direct mail [6]. This may be because physicians find personal sources of information (i.e., with a PCR) more credible than nonpersonal sources such as advertisements in medical journals [7].

A Critical Approach to the "Detailing" Interaction

PCRs perform a function that is appreciated. They visit at the physician's convenience and provide information in a friendly and positive manner [3]. Nonetheless the need for physicians to be more critical of the detailing process has been highlighted [3, 10, 11].

Franko et al. [11] describe promotional techniques such as "fallacies in logic" that can lead us to invalid conclusions. Organizations have used "counterdetailing" approaches [12], where pharmacy faculty discuss the pharmacokinetics, therapeutic usefulness and side effects of the promoted "drug of the day." Academic detailing [13–15] has also been described, in which faculty travel to visit clinicians for face-to-face discussions using educational reminders and prescriber profiling. Although such exercises yield positive effects on prescriber behaviors, they are costly and time-consuming interventions. (For more details, please refer to Chapter 5.)

Summary

☐ Detailing of physicians by PCRs remains a frequent occurrence in medical settings.
☐ PCRs provide an efficient way of obtaining information about new medications.
☐ Prescribing behaviors influenced by detailing activities may be nonrational and expensive.
☐ Physicians need to become more critical in their interactions with PCRs to ensure they are prescribing based on scientific data and good clinical rationale as opposed to PI promotion.

References

1. Barton L. Ethics, profit and patients. When pharmaceutical companies sponsor medical meetings. J Hosp Mark 1993; 8(1):71–82

2. Gaedeke RM, Tootlelian DH, Sanders EE. Value of services provided by pharmaceutical companies: Perceptions of physicians and pharmaceutical sales representatives. Health Mark Q 1999; 17(1):23–31

3. Ferguson RP. Need for better interactions between physicians and pharmaceutical sales representatives. Ann Pharmacother 2002; 36(12): 1966–8

4. Ferguson RP, Rhim E, Belizaire W, Egede L, Carter K, Larsdale T. Encounters with pharmaceutical sales representatives among practicing internists. Am J Med 1999; 107(2):149–52

5. Ma J, Stafford RS, Cockburn IM, Finkelstein SN. A statistical analysis of the magnitude and composition of drug promotion in the US in 1998. Clin Ther 2003; 25(5):1503–17

6. Manchanda P, Honka E. The effects and role of direct to physician marketing in the pharmaceutical industry: An integrative review. Yale J Health Policy Law Ethics 2005; 5(2):785–822

7. Spiller LD, Wymer WW. Physicians' perceptions and uses of commercial drug information sources: An examination of pharmaceutical marketing to physicians. Health Mark Q 2001; 19(1):91–106

8. Greene JA. Attention to "details": Etiquette and the pharmaceutical salesman in postwar America. Soc Stud Sci 2004; 34(2):271–92

9. Wazana A. Physicians and the pharmaceutical industry. Is a gift ever just a gift? JAMA 2000; 283(3):373–80

10. Ferguson RP. Training the resident to meet the detail men. JAMA 1989; 261(7):992–3

11. Franko JP, Shaughnessey AF, Slawson DC. Obtaining useful information from pharmaceutical company representatives. In: *Information Mastery: Evidence Based Family Medicine*, 2nd ed. (WW Rosser, DC Slawson and AF Shaughnessy, Eds.). BC Decker, 2004

12. Levinson W, Dunn PM. Counterdetailing. JAMA 1984; 251(16):2084

13. Siegel D, Lopez J, Meier J, Goldstein MK, Lee S, Brazill BJ, Matalka MS. Academic detailing to improve antihypertensive prescribing patterns. Am J Hypertens 2003; 16(6):508–11

14. Denton GD, Smith J, Faust J, Holmboe E. Comparing the efficacy of staff versus housestaff instruction in an intervention to improve hypertension management. Acad Med 2001; 76(12):1257–60

15. Moser SE, Dorsch JN, Kellerman R. The RAFT approach to academic detailing with preceptors. Fam Med 2004; 36(5):316–18

4 Medical Academia and the Pharmaceutical Industry

Bob was feeling happy. He had just received the prescriber profiling information that he had requested. It appeared sales of Vivre had gone up after the dinner talk last week. Bob had expected this. The speaker, Dr. Johnson, an eminent academic psychiatrist, was employed by MedCorp to give talks on Vivre. He was a charismatic, much respected clinician with an impeccable CV. He had been involved in the company-sponsored trials for Vivre and had been impressed by the medication. Subsequently, he had become involved in doing many industry-sponsored educational activities for the medication. Dr. Johnson was paid for his time and received tens of thousands of dollars a year in additional income from these activities. Having seen the encouraging figures, Bob called Dr. Johnson to arrange several more speaking engagements over the coming months.

U.S. academic centers have partnered with industry so that academic innovation can be rapidly and efficiently brought to market [1]. Concerns have been raised that academia is no longer as autonomous as it once was and that industry sponsorship may influence the outcome of research and undermine traditionally held academic values [1–3].

Examples of academic institutions' relationships with private industry include ownership of stock in the sponsors of research being conducted at the institution and specific research centers and teaching programs in which students and faculty members essentially carry out industry research [1, 4, 5].

On an individual basis, academic employees (e.g., Institutional Review Board [IRB] members and institutional decision makers) may have significant ties with industry. Researchers may receive research support through grants, may receive fees for supporting marketing activities, or may receive honoraria for speaking on behalf of industry [1, 4, 5].

Jane was waiting for her 3:00 P.M. weekly supervision meeting with Dr. Johnson. She always looked forward to this time; Dr. Johnson was a respected professor with an excellent reputation and was a very effective teacher. Jane valued this time to discuss the psychiatric cases that she was seeing as part of her mental health elective. Today she wanted to learn when she should use certain types of antidepressants; there seemed to be so many available on the market and she often felt confused as to which one to use when.

Dr. Johnson reviewed the different antidepressants available on the market and their different indications with Jane. Jane asked him about his personal preferences. He talked about Vivre and why he liked it so much; he had enrolled 20 patients as part of a multicentered drug trial and liked the results. He also told Jane he was confident that Vivre could be used for other disorders such as panic disorder and that he had had some success with his own patients. Jane asked whether Vivre had an FDA indication for use in panic disorder. Dr. Johnson said that it did not, but it would only be a matter of time before it did.

Researchers have argued that industry–academia relationships should only be permitted when there is legitimate justification for them [1]. Some go even further to assert that academic medical centers

(AMCs) must strongly regulate and in some cases prohibit many common practices that constitute conflicts of interest with drug and medical device companies [4, 5]. The Association of American Medical Colleges (AAMC) has recommended general safeguards and institutional procedures for the management of academic commercial ties.

Commercial Influence Over the Process of Scientific Publication

The increasing influence of industry on medical research has persuaded editors of medical journals to agree on strict rules governing authors reporting sponsorship and conflicts of interest [6, 7]. Concerns regarding conflict of interest also extend to editors, with some journals requesting that editors should divest themselves of financial ties with industry on assuming editorial duties [8, 9].

Use of ghost authors, that is, industry-paid professional writers who are employed directly by the PI or medical education communication companies (MECCs), has also generated controversy [2]. Their contribution to a paper may vary, but includes writing a first draft or editing a paper written by authors [9]. (They are not named as authors.) Critics have argued that this practice might undermine accountability and bias the paper's content [11]. Journal editors have pointed out that it is absolutely unacceptable to represent as one's own scholarly work the prepared work of pharmaceutical companies' contract writers [12]. Studies investigating the effect of professional writers on authorship note that industry-coordinated papers were, on average, cited more frequently in the literature, published in journals with a higher "impact factor" and authored by academics with more Medline listed publications [13]. Suggested solutions to this problem include encouraging good practice [10], that is, disclosing professional writers' contributions in a specific manner.

In addition, studies have shown that lead authors of scientific publications and clinical practice guidelines (CPGs) frequently have financial conflicts of interest that are directly relevant to the content of the publication [14, 15].

Medical journals themselves receive substantial income from the PI in the form of industry purchasing of advertising, reprints and sponsorship of supplements. Furthermore, free publications sent to physicians are completely dependent on income from pharmaceutical advertising [16].

Pharmaceutical Industry and Clinical Research Trials

Seventy percent of financial support for clinical drug trials in the United States comes from industry rather than from the National Institutes of Health (NIH) [11]. Industry currently spends approximately $3.5 billion annually to conduct trials in the United States [17]. As a result, financial conflicts of interest in clinical research have grown more important for investigators and institutions alike [18]. Pharmaceutical industry–funded research takes place not only in academic medical centers but also in commercially operated (i.e., for-profit) networks of contract research organizations (CROs) and site management organizations (SMOs) [11, 19].

Examples of ethical issues raised in industry-sponsored clinical research include erosion of informed consent procedures, compromise of patient confidentiality and enrollment of ineligible subjects [19].

Significant research efforts have been dedicated to analyzing the reliability of data acquired from industry-sponsored trials. Examples include modifications of traditional study design such as enrolling study participants with milder disease or who are healthier than the population who will actually receive the drug [11]; using a dose of the comparable drug that is outside of the standard clinical range; using misleading research measurement scales; and statistical obfuscation [20]. All of these methods can be used to present study results in a more favorable light for the sponsor.

Actual study data is generally stored centrally, with investigators receiving only portions, and this has raised concerns regarding excessive control of trial data by industry [10]. Bias in publication (e.g., repeatedly publishing the same or similar findings for impact; selectively highlighting findings favorable to the sponsor and withholding unfavorable results) has also been emphasized [21–4]. In particular, multiple publications of the same information leading to overestimation of the efficacy of an intervention highlight how data can artificially skew balance of opinion in favor of a new drug [25].

More recently, the concept of registration of clinical trials highlights worries over publication bias (i.e., scientists publishing positive findings more often than negative findings), and the potential that such bias will harm trust between patient and investigator has led to researchers advocating a comprehensive mandatory registration of clinical trials [26–8]. In September 2004, leading medical journals announced that they would require, as a condition of consideration for publication, registration in a public trials registry.

Summary

□ U.S. academic medical centers have become closely linked with the pharmaceutical industry.
□ Medical editors and authors of scientific papers should disclose financial ties with industry that pose a potential conflict of interest.
□ Medical journals themselves receive substantial income from the pharmaceutical industry.
□ Manipulation of scientific data (e.g., withholding negative trial data, multiple publication of the same data) has led to a call for the mandatory registration of all clinical trials.

References

1. Johns MM, Barnes M, Florencio PS. Restoring balance to industry–academia relationships in an era of institutional financial conflicts of interest: Promoting research while maintaining trust. JAMA 2003; 289(6):741–6

2. Brodkey AC. The role of the pharmaceutical industry in teaching psychopharmacology: A growing problem. Acad Psychiatry 2005; 29(2):222–9

3. Boyd EA, Bero LA. Assessing faculty financial relationships with industry: A case study. JAMA 2000; 284(17):2209–14

4. Angell M. Is academic medicine for sale? N Engl J Med 2000; 342(20): 1516–18

5. Brennan TA, Rothman DJ, Blank L, Blumenthal D, Chimonas SC, Cohen JJ, Goldman J, Kassirer JP, Kimball H, Naughton J, Smelser A. Health industry practices that create conflicts of interest. JAMA 2006; 295(4):429–33

6. Davidoff F. Between the lines: Navigating the uncharted territory of industry-sponsored research. Health Aff (Millwood) 2002; 21(2):235–42

7. Davidoff F, DeAngelis CD, Drazen JM, Hoey J, Hojgaard L, Horton R, et al. Sponsorship, authorship, and accountability. Lancet 2001; 358:854–6

8. Wright IC. Conflict of interest and the British Journal of Psychiatry. Br J Psychiatry 2002; 180:82–3

9. Just how tainted has medicine become? [Editorial]. Lancet 2002; 359:1167–8

10. Lagnado M. Increasing the trust in scientific authorship. Br J Psychiatry 2003; 183:3–4

11. Bodenheimer T. Uneasy alliance – clinical investigators and the pharmaceutical industry. N Engl J Med 2000; 342(20):1539–44

12. Rae-Grant Ø. Challenges of the pharmaceutical–physician boundary. Can J Psychiatry 2003; 48(5):287–8

13. Healy D, Cattell D. Interface between authorship: Industry and science in the domain of therapeutics. Br J Psychiatry 2003; 183:22–7

14. Krimsky S, Rothenberg LS, Stott P, Kyle G. Scientific journals and their authors' financial interests. Psychother Psychosom 1998; 67(4–5): 194–201

15. Choudhry NK, Stelfox HT, Detsky AS. Relationships between authors of clinical practice guidelines and the pharmaceutical industry. JAMA 2002; 287(5):612–17

16. Smith R. Medical journals and pharmaceutical companies: Uneasy bedfellows. BMJ 2003: 326(7400):1202–5

17. Ashar BH, Miller RG, Getz KJ, Powe NR. Prevalence and determinants of physician participation in conducting pharmaceutical-sponsored clinical trials and lectures. J Gen Intern Med 2004; 19(11):1140–5

18. Warner TD, Roberts LW. Scientific integrity; fidelity and conflicts of interest in research. Curr Opin Psychiatry 2004; 17:381–5

19. Mirowski P, Van Horn R. The contract research organization and the commercialization of scientific research. Soc Stud Sci 2005; 35(4):503–48

20. Puttagunta PS, Caulfield TA, Griener G. Conflict of interest in clinical research. Health Law Rev 2002; 10(2):30–2

21. Safer DJ. Design and reporting modifications in industry-sponsored comparative psychopharmacology trials. J Nerv Ment Dis 2002; 190(9):583–92

22. Baker CB, Johnsrud MT, Crismon ML, Rosenheck RA, Woods SW. Quantitative analysis of sponsorship bias in economic studies of antidepressants. Br J Psychiatry 2003; 183:498–506

23. Melander H, Ahlquist-Rastad J, Meijer G, Beerman B. Evidence b(i)ased medicine. BMJ 2003: 326(7400):1171–3

24. Lexchin J, Bero LA, Djulbegovic B, Clark O. Pharmaceutical industry sponsorship and research outcome and quality: Systematic review. BMJ 2003; 326(7400):1167–70

25. Rennie D. Fair conduct and fair reporting of clinical trials. JAMA 1999; 282(18):1766–8

26. Dickersin K, Rennie D. Registering clinical trials. JAMA 2003; 290(4):516–23

27. Steinbrook R. Registration of clinical trials – voluntary or mandatory? N Engl J Med 2004; 351(18):1820–2

28. Rennie D. Trial registration: A great idea switches from ignored to irresistible. JAMA 2004; 292(11):1359–62

5 Teaching Physicians in Training about Pharmaceutical Industry Promotion

Jack briefed his medical team on the management of Mrs. Bratton's hyponatremia. They all congregated outside her room on the corridor of a busy teaching hospital. Jack was enjoying being a chief resident, especially his time as an attending when he could teach. After rounds, Jack sat writing some notes. The exhausted post call team sitting around him broke into conversation... last night's football scores; the latest hospital gossip; what to have for dinner. "Hey, I know," said the senior resident, Craig. "The MedCorp rep told me to call him if we ever wanted to go out for dinner... he told me he'd take us to Zucci's." Craig picked up the phone and minutes later had arranged for the whole team to be taken out to one of the most expensive restaurants in the city. "Dr. Jones, are you coming?" asked Craig as they all headed out. Jack smiled uneasily. "No, I don't think so, guys... you go have fun." As he watched his team file out, Jack sat back and thought about what had just happened. His team had worked hard and done a good job, but he wondered if, as their teacher and supervisor, it was okay for him to sanction their free dinner.

Medical students have extensive exposure to pharmaceutical industry marketing during their early years of training [1]. The need to educate physicians in training about PPII and PI promotion (i.e., to increase their promotional literacy) has been highlighted by researchers [2–5]. Despite this and professional guidelines [6,7], recent studies show that physicians remain permissive in their views about a variety of PI marketing activities [8]. In addition, physicians [9] and medical students [10] continue to demonstrate low levels of knowledge about PPII in general. Furthermore, few curricula exist that address PPII [9].

In 2002 the Accreditation Council for Graduate Medical Education (ACGME) published a paper on this very issue [7].

> The conflict of values between the professional ethics of the physician and the business ethics of industry is impossible to ignore. Nowhere is this conflict more apparent than in the conduct of promotional activities. . . . It is the chief means by which industry relates to physicians, residents and medical students.

Following is a summary of ACGME recommendations on what trainees should learn about PPII:

☐ Residents must learn how promotional activities can influence judgment in prescribing decisions and research activities

☐ Residents must understand the purpose, development and application of drug formularies and clinical guidelines

☐ Resident curricula should include how to apply appropriate considerations of cost-benefit analysis as a component of prescribing practice

☐ Resident curricular should include discussion and reflection on managing encounters with industry representatives

Illustrative cases of how to handle patient requests for medication, particularly with regard to Direct to Consumer Advertising of drugs, should be included in communication skills curricula. (ACGME: Principles to Guide the Relationship between Graduate Medical Education and Industry. September 10, 2002.)

> Jack sat in the faculty meeting, nervously checking his watch. The meeting was getting heated, with the department chair very

upset. "This behavior is outrageous...the residents are averaging $150 per week each in benefits from drug reps."

"How did you come up with that figure?" asked Dr. Chadwick, a senior faculty member.

"When you average the cost of freebies, meals, speaker honoraria, that's what you get. This has gotten out of control...whatever happened to professionalism?" exclaimed the chairman. Jack sighed; his junior status at the meeting stopped him from speaking his mind. He looked at the chairman – in his late 60's, a formidable figure, opinionated, confident and distinguished – and thought, "I wonder how much debt he graduated with? He doesn't get it. Medicine isn't what it was like 30 years ago.... A free meal at a fancy restaurant is one of the perks – that's all, a perk."

"Jack, what do you think?" Jack's daydream was interrupted by his chair's booming voice. "You must be up on all the ACGME and AMA policies about this stuff. What are you teaching the residents about this?"

Jack's face reddened and his pulse quickened as he realized he had no idea what the chairman was referring to. "Um...sure, I can look into it," he mumbled.

How to Teach Tomorrow's Physicians about PI Promotion

This topic often generates heated debate among physicians [2], who may show disbelief and hostility at the suggestion that their medical judgment can be influenced by the pharmaceutical industry [11]. Also, there is often a "self-serving bias": Students are more likely to see the influence of PI enticements on others' behavior than their own [12]. In view of these resistances, innovative methods used to teach medical ethics topics, such as case-based exercises, group discussion and the use of standardized patients, may be useful [13]. Resident and faculty interviewed expressed a preference for small-group and panel discussion, lecture series and critical reading skills seminars as preferred methods to teach this topic [9]. Several such curricula have been reported in the literature [4, 5, 9, 11, 14–22].

Specific Teaching Strategies Used to Teach about PPII with Demonstrated Efficacy

- ☐ Patient interviews about their experience with costly prescription medications [9]
- ☐ Faculty-led debate and discussion of relevant academic literature [17]
- ☐ Using critical interpretation skills to evaluate promotional material [9, 11, 15, 16, 22]
- ☐ Group critiquing of promotional materials, such as advertisements in medical journals [4, 5, 9, 11, 14–16, 22]
- ☐ Teaching about the policies of medical professional societies [9, 11]
- ☐ Evidence-facilitated debate: "Would pharmaceutical companies subsidize marketing methods if they were not rewarding?" [11]
- ☐ Post-PCR analysis of presentation; faculty observation of resident interviews with PCRs [5, 11, 15, 16, 22]
- ☐ Discussion by pharmacy faculty of the pharmacokinetics, therapeutic usefulness and side effects of the promoted "drug of the day" [5, 18, 19]
- ☐ Faculty travel to clinicians for face-to-face discussions with use of educational reminders and prescriber profiling [19–21]

The aim of most curricula has been to help physicians in training develop an informed approach to their interactions with PCRs or the PI. A useful concept introduced by Shaughnessey et al. [5] is to train physicians to "function more as information managers and not just information repositories," hence challenging the historically passive stance physicians have in encounters with PCRs.

Anastasio and Little [17] developed a checklist of questions for residents to use during interactions with PCRs:

- ☐ What is your educational and professional background?
- ☐ How long have you been with your company?
- ☐ What products does your company have? What are you planning on talking about today?
- ☐ How does your new product compare with Drug X which is what I usually prescribe for this condition?
- ☐ What are the drug's adverse effects? How many patients discontinue the drug? What types of patients should not take the drug?
- ☐ How much does this medication cost per month (or course) at our local pharmacy? How does this compare with Drug X that I normally prescribe?
- ☐ Can you name a well-controlled drug study which compares your new drug with others frequently prescribed for the same condition?

(Republished with the permission of *Pharmacotherapy*.)

Shaughnessey et al. [5] differentiate between rational reasons to use a drug, such as greater effectiveness, patient convenience and lower cost, and nonrational appeals used by PCRs during drug detailing. Examples of the latter include appealing to authority ("Dr.——— uses my drug"), the bandwagon effect ("Everyone is using this drug"), the red herring (giving factual but irrelevant data) and the challenge ("Prove me wrong by trying my drug"). Increasing trainee awareness of such strategies can help increase their promotional literacy.

Summary

- ☐ Medical trainees need to be taught about PPII.
- ☐ Widespread naiveté persists among trainees and faculty about the medical literature and professional policies on this topic.

☐ Studies testing the effectiveness of educational interventions have been encouraging.

☐ This topic often generates heated debate among physicians.

References

1. Bellin M, McCarthy S, Drevlow L, Pierach C. Medical students' exposure to pharmaceutical industry marketing: A survey of one U.S. medical school. Acad Med 2004; 79(11):1041–5

2. Wazana A.Physicians and the pharmaceutical industry. Is a gift ever just a gift? JAMA 2000; 283(3):373–80

3. Kassirer JP. Financial indigestion. JAMA 2000; 284(17):2156–7

4. Ferguson RP. Training the resident to meet the detail men. JAMA 1989; 261(7):992–3

5. Shaughnessy AF, Slawson DC, Bennett JH. Teaching information mastery: Evaluating information provided by pharmaceutical representatives. Fam Med 1995; 27(9):581–5

6. American Medical Association Council on Ethical and Judicial Affairs. Opinion 8.0601: Gifts to physicians from industry. Available at: http://www.ama-assn.org/ama/pub/category/4001.html (last accessed June 2006)

7. Principles to guide the relationship between graduate medical education and industry. Available at: http://www.acgme.org (under GME information; under Position Papers; last accessed June 2006). Accreditation Council for Graduate Medical Education, 2002

8. Brett AS, Burr W, Moloo J. Are gifts from pharmaceutical companies ethically problematic? Arch Intern Med 2003; 163(18):2213–18

9. Watkins RS, Kimberly J Jr. What residents don't know about physician pharmaceutical industry interactions. Acad Med 2004; 79(5):432–7

10. Monaghan MS, Galt KA, Turner PD, Houghton BL, Rich EC, Markert RJ, Bergman-Evans B. Student understanding of the relationship between the health professions and the pharmaceutical industry. Teach Learn Med 2003; 15(1):14–20

11. Wilkes MS, Hoffman JR. An innovative approach to educating medical students about pharmaceutical promotion. Acad Med 2001 Dec; 76(12):1271–7

12. Dana J, Loewenstein G. A social science perspective on gifts to physicians from industry. JAMA 2003; 290(2):252–5

13. Smith S, Fryer-Edwards K, Diekema DS, Braddock CH 3rd. Finding effective strategies for teaching medical ethics: A comparison trial of two interventions. Acad Med 2004; 79(3):265–71

14. Hopper JA, Speece MW, Musial JL. Effects of an educational intervention on residents' knowledge and attitudes toward interactions with pharmaceutical representatives. J Gen Intern Med 1997; 12(10):639–42

15. Palmisano P, Edelstein J. Teaching drug promotion abuses to health profession students. J Med Educ 1980; 55(5):453–5

16. Anastasio GD, Little JM Jr. Pharmaceutical marketing: Implications for medical residency training. Pharmacotherapy 1996; 16(1):103–7

17. Agrawal S, Saluja I, Kaczorowski J. A prospective before and after trial of an educational intervention about pharmaceutical marketing. Acad Med 2004; 79(11):1046–50

18. Levinson W, Dunn PM. Counterdetailing. JAMA 1984; 251(16):2084

19. Siegel D, Lopez J, Meier J, Goldstein M, KLee S, Brazill BJ, Matalka MS. Academic detailing to improve antihypertensive prescribing patterns. Am J Hypertens 2003; 16(6):508–11

20. Denton GD, Smith J, Faust J, Holmboe E. Comparing the efficacy of staff versus house staff instruction in an intervention to improve hypertension management. Acad Med 2001; 76(12):1257–60

21. Moser SE, Dorsch JN, Kellerman R. The RAFT approach to academic detailing with preceptors. Fam Med 2004; 36(5):316–18

22. Kelcher S, Brownoff R, Meadows LM. Structured approach to pharmaceutical representatives. Can Fam Physician 1998; 44:1053–60

6 Continuing Medical Education

How to Separate Continuing Medical Education from Pharmaceutical Industry Promotion

---

Jane checked her watch. She was post call and on rounds; the grand rounds she had planned to attend had already started. The speaker was Dr. Bow, a professor from a prestigious medical school who was an expert on mood disorders. Jane had read his book focusing on pharmacological management of mood disorders and had been looking forward to hearing him speak.

Continuing medical education (CME) is critically important for physicians to keep abreast of the latest developments in patient care [1]. In response to congressional investigation of questionable pharmaceutical marketing practices of the 1980's, the American Medical Association and six other groups formed the Accreditation Council for Continuing Medical Education (ACCME) [2]. The ACCME's 1992 "Standards for Commercial Support" sets forth norms that govern the professional relationships between commercial interests and continuing medical education providers [3]. The need for such statements arises from the fact that year after year, the major pharmaceutical companies invest millions to support educational activities developed and certified by accredited CME providers [2].

The ACCME defines commercial bias as "favoring one product over another in a manner that is perceived to be or intended to advance the commercial interest of the product, device or service that physicians control, use, deploy or manage in the care of patients" [3]. Concerns over the presence of commercial bias in CME have sparked much debate in the academic literature. In 2004 [3] the ACCME and ACGME presented a joint statement, which said, in part, that "commercial bias is prohibited across the continuum of medical education." Nonetheless, concern has been expressed that product promotion and not medical education is the objective of industry-sponsored education [4–6] and that commercial bias in CME settings has the potential to affect independent judgment of medical professionals [1, 7].

Later, as she headed out to the hospital car park, Jane met Bob from MedCorp. His company had sponsored the grand rounds that morning, and he asked Jane if she had been there. Jane expressed her regrets at missing the lecture. Bob produced a leaflet from his briefcase; it was an invitation to a dinner talk with Dr. Bow that very evening. Jane happily took the flier and thanked Bob; she would most definitely be there to hear the respected doctor speak.

The Advantages and Disadvantages of Industry Support for CME

Promotion by industry frequently occurs through financial support for a broad array of educational programs [3, 6]. According to ACCME's report, more than half of the funding for the CME enterprise came from commercial support [8]. The commercial role is expected to grow as new, for-profit medical education communication companies (MECCs) also provide CME [6].

Advantages of Industry Support for CME

☐ Public funding for CME is relatively inadequate [2].
☐ Industry is an abundant source of advances in medicine and technology, and its desire to quickly disperse information about its products helps to fill an important need [9].
☐ The pharmaceutical industry (PI) is serving a mutual interest with physicians to ensure that patients receive the most up-to-date and appropriate care [2].

Disadvantages of Industry Support for CME

☐ The presence of commercial bias; for example, educational articles and meeting reports sponsored by industry are not externally vetted and can be advertising disguised as educational material [10].
☐ Skewing of topics to favor "treatment" or "medical management" of illness rather than diagnosis, and so forth [11, 12].
☐ Industry-supported educational activities are slanted in favor of the source of financial support, and physicians attending such courses later prescribe those products more often than the competing drug [13].
☐ Finally, there is the concern that the institution of medicine could be perceived as an extension of the PI with subsequent erosion of trust in the profession [5].

Jane arrived at the restaurant and was greeted by the maitre d' and taken to the table. Bob was there and was sitting next to Dr. Bow. There were a few attendees, who chatted informally through a variety of mouth-watering appetizers. Dr. Bow began his talk after the expensive entrees had been ordered. Jane could not help but notice how often Dr. Bow mentioned Vivre, and his talk seemed to be more focused on this. She left the meal disappointed in the quality of the talk.

Indicators of High-Quality CME

□ When faculty or speakers must use trade names in a GME or CME presentation, they should cite similar products or services of several companies rather than focusing on a single supporting company [1, 14].

□ The budget for the event should be controlled by the provider of the CME so social activities do not compete with the educational event [1].

□ The provider of CME should ban the distribution of promotional materials in educational sessions [1, 3].

□ Disclosure of commercial support should be provided to registrants in general program materials [1, 3].

□ Ultimate decisions on organization, content and choice of CME should lie with physician organizers [3, 14].

Suggested Techniques to Further Enhance the Quality of CME

□ Manufacturers should not be permitted to provide supports directly to any ACCME-accredited program. Instead, they should contribute to a central repository, which in turn would distribute the funds [12, 15, 16].

□ Faculty, deans and program directors should also promote sensitivity to potential biases by providing specific education to help trainees evaluate industry programs and information [1, 11].

□ Providers of CME must also control access to registrants' mailing addresses [1].

□ The definition of "full disclosure" should be broadened; that is, industry should indicate full the amount they have contributed to programming [11].

Promotional Programs versus CME: What's the Difference?

Promotional	CME
FDA/DDMAC – regulated as part of the sale of medicine	ACCME – regulated as part of the practice of medicine
PDR LABEL	*Balance!*
Single drug is the focus	Unmet needs of the practitioner are the focus
Pharma company is responsible for content	Accredited provider (educational institute) is responsible for content and is NOT an agent of the company
Commercial pharma sponsor is direct payer to speaker and chooses faculty	Pharma is third-party payer (educational grant to accredited provider who chooses faculty)
Speaker is an agent of the pharma company	Speaker is not an agent of the pharma company
	May be multiply sponsored

Table taken from Stahl S. It takes two to entangle. Clin Psychiatry News 2005 (March). Reproduced with permission of NEI Press. ISBN: 1553–8915 (online); 1553–8907 (print). Available online at www.neiglobal.com.

Stahl [17] highlights the need to disentangle educational activities aimed at optimizing medical practices from promotional activities aimed at optimizing pharmaceutical sales. (See Table 6.1.)

References

1. Coyle SL. Physician–industry relations. Part 2: Organizational issues. Ann Intern Med 2002; 136(5):403–6
2. Wilson FS. Continuing medical education: Ethical collaboration between sponsor and industry. Clin Orthop 2003; (412):33–7

3. ACGME and ACCME. Joint statement regarding graduate and continuing medical education's relationship with industry. November 2004

4. Capozzi JD, Rhodes R, Delsignore J. Medical education and corporate sponsorship. J Bone Joint Surg Am 2003; 85A(1):168–70

5. Packer S, Parke DW. Ethical concerns in industry support of CME. Arch Ophthalmol 2004; 122(5):773–6

6. Relman AS. Separating continuing medical education from pharmaceutical marketing. JAMA 2001; 285(15):2009–12

7. Tenery RM Jr. Interactions between physicians and the health care technology industry. JAMA 2000; 283(3):391–3

8. *Accreditation Council for Continuing Medical Education Annual Report Data 2001.* ACCME, Chicago, 2002

9. Holmer AF. Industry strongly supports continuing medical education. JAMA 2001; 285(15):2012–14

10. Chepesiuk R. Supported by an unrestricted educational grant. CMAJ 2003; 169 (5):421–2

11. Davis DA. CME and the pharmaceutical industry: Two worlds, three views, four steps. CMAJ 2004; 171(2):149–50

12. Katz HP, Goldfinger SE, Fletcher SW. Academia industry collaboration in continuing medical education: Description of two approaches. J Contin Educ Health Prof 2002; 22(1):43–54

13. Bowman MA, Pearle DL. Changes in drug prescribing patterns related to commercial company funding of continuing medical education. J Contin Educ Health Prof 1988; 8(1):13–20

14. CMA policy summary. Physicians and the pharmaceutical industry. CMAJ 1994; 256A–C

15. Brennan TA, Rothman DJ, Blank L, Blumenthal D, Chimonas SC, Cohen JJ, Goldman J, Kassirer JP, Kimball H, Naughton J, Smelser N. Health industry practices that create conflicts of interest. JAMA 2006; 295(4):429–33

16. Lexchin J, Cassels A. Does the C in CME stand for "continuing" or "commercial"? CMAJ, 2005; 172(2):160–2

17. Stahl S. It takes two to entangle: Separating medical education from pharmaceutical promotion. Psychopharmacology Educational Update. 2005 (March):1, 6

7 Professional Policies on Physician–Pharmaceutical Industry Interaction (PPII)

In recent decades many professional organizations have produced ethical guidelines or position statements on PPII. These documents cover many areas of interactions, from accepting gifts or continuing medical education (CME) support to conducting ethical research collaborations.

The American Medical Association (AMA) responded to public concerns regarding PPII in the 1980's with a code of medical ethics recommending that gifts to physicians should benefit patients, relate to the physician's work and be of minimal value [1].

Concern about increases in pharmaceutical industry (PI) promotion in training settings led to a 2002 position paper from the Accreditation Committee for Graduate Medical Education (ACGME) that emphasized the need to separate medical education from PI promotion [2].

The Accreditation Council for Continuing Medical Education (ACCME) has six standards for commercial support of CME activities [3].

The Association of American Medical Colleges has issued a publication in 2 parts titled Protecting Subjects, Preserving Trust and Promoting Progress [4, 5].

The evidence of PI influence on medicine and the ensuing concern for professional integrity and patient care resulted in the American College of Physicians – American Society of Internal Medicine producing two ethical position papers [6, 7]. Both papers cover PI gifts to physicians; PI influence on medical education; academic and industry collaboration; and influence on medical professional societies.

In 1994 the Canadian Medical Association published a position paper, "Physicians and the Pharmaceutical Industry." Guidelines were developed by the CMA to assist physicians in determining when a relationship with industry is appropriate [8]. The guidelines cover areas such as industry-sponsored research, support for CME and provision of samples. They also highlight the importance of medical school curricula that "deal explicitly with the guidelines."

Without exception, all these guidelines establish that it is unethical for physicians to accept gifts or support in any form that results in recommendation of a particular product or delivery of a particular clinical action [2].

In addition to these guidelines, many residency programs, teaching hospitals and medical specialties have their own regulations [9–11].

Voluntary codes of conduct for industry developed by the Pharmaceutical Research and Manufacturers of America were adopted in 2002 [12]. With a primary focus on PI marketing activities, most prohibit companies from giving doctors inducements to prescribe their products in the form of payments, lavish gifts or extravagant hospitality [13, 14]. The American Academy of Pharmaceutical Physicians also has a brief Code of Ethics [15].

The Office of the Inspector General (OIG) of the U.S. Department of Health and Human Services issued guidelines to pharmaceutical manufacturers for developing programs to ensure legal compliance [16]. In addition, HIPAA, the U.S. Federal Health Insurance Portability and Accountability Act, has altered the physician's relationship with pharmaceutical company representatives (PCRs) [17].

The advantage of setting such policies is that such efforts aim to clearly articulate and concretize ethical principles [18]. Disadvantages of such policies include limitations in interpretation; also, the policies are ineffective unless actively promoted by organizations or training programs, and many policies lack specificity about the kinds of relationships that are actually permitted [9, 12, 18].

(Refer to Appendix I for full versions of some of the policies just outlined.)

References

1. American Medical Association Council on Ethical and Judicial Affairs. Opinion 8.061: Gifts to -physicians from industry. Available at: http://www.ama-assn.org/ama/pub/category/4001.html (last accessed June 2006)

2. Principles to guide the relationship between graduate medical education and industry. Available at: http://www.acgme.org (under GME information; under position papers) (last accessed June 2006). ACGME, 2002

3. http://www.accme.org "Ask ACCME" http://www.accme.org/index.cfm/fa/faq.home/Faq.cfm Refer to the six standards of commercial support. Last accessed 12/2006

4. AAMC Task Force on Financial Conflicts of Interest in Clinical Research. Protecting subjects, preserving trust, promoting progress: Policy and guidelines for the oversight of individual financial interests in human subjects research. Association of American Medical Colleges, 2001. Available at: www.aamc.org/research/coi/start.htm (last accessed June 2006)

5. AAMC Task Force on Financial Conflicts of Interest in Clinical Research. Protecting subjects, preserving trust, promoting progress II: Principles and recommendations for oversight of an institution's financial interests in human subjects research. Association of American Medical Colleges, 2002. Available at: www.aamc.org/research/coi/start.htm (last accessed June 2006)

6. Coyle SL. Physician–industry relations, part 1: Individual physicians. Ann Intern Med 2002; 136(5):396–402

7. Coyle SL. Physician–industry relations, part 2: Organizational issues. Ann Intern Med 2002; 136(5):403–6

8. CMA Policy Summary. Physicians and the pharmaceutical industry. CMAJ 1994; 150:256A–C. Available at: http://www.cma.ca (under policy/advocacy; under CMA policy base) (last accessed June 2006)

9. Wazana A, Granich A, Primeau F, Bhanji, NH, Jalbert M. Using the literature in developing McGill's guidelines for interactions between residents and the pharmaceutical industry. Acad Med 2004; 79(11):1033–40

10. Whal DS, American Psychiatric Association Ethics Committee. Ethics Primer of the American Psychiatric Association. APA, 2001

11. American College of Obstetricians and Gynecologists. Guidelines for relationships with industry. Obstet Gynecol 2001; 98(4):703–6

12. Tsai AC. Policies to regulate gifts to physicians from industry. JAMA 2003; 290:1776

13. Wager E. How to dance with porcupines: Rules and guidelines on doctors' relations with drug companies. BMJ 2003 Aug 9; 327(7410):341

14. Code for interactions with health care professionals) http://www.phrma.org/code_on_interactions_with_healthcare_professionals/ Last accessed 12/2006

15. American Academy of Pharmaceutical Physicians. Code of ethics. Available at: www.aapp.org/ethics.php (last accessed June 2006)

16. Office of Inspector General. Compliance Program Guidance for Pharmaceutical Manufacturers. Available at: www.oig.hhs.gov/fraud/complianceguidance.html (last accessed June 2006)

17. American Medical Association. Interactions with pharmaceutical industry representatives. Available at: http://www.ama-assn.org/ama/pub/category/11910.html (last accessed June 2006)

18. Mohl PC. Psychiatric training program engagement with the pharmaceutical industry: An educational issue, not strictly an ethical one. Acad Psychiatry 2005; 29(2):215–21

8 Preserving Professionalism

Patients' Perceptions of

Physicians' Acceptance of Gifts

from the Pharmaceutical Industry

As Bob settled into the chair in the waiting room, he was worried about the email he'd received from his boss that morning. The company was facing a major lawsuit over the emergence of severe side effects from a well-prescribed medication. In preparation for the suit the company is making extensive budget cuts. The pressure was on to improve performance in all departments. Bob had been with the company for two decades. He loved his job, especially the "people" aspect of it, but the job was becoming increasingly stressful, with more and more pressure to increase sales. Considering alimony payments and his eldest son heading for college, Bob knew that losing his job would be disastrous. Bob sat in the waiting room of the hospital mental health services clinic in the hope of catching Dr. Jensan in between patients. Bob wanted to follow up with her about the dinner his company had sponsored the night before with a prominent speaker. Bob had found that following up was a good way of asking physicians about their opinions of his company's new antidepressant medication, Vivre. The clinic receptionist appeared, so Bob walked over to chat. He also had invitations for a company-sponsored luncheon at Zucci's he wanted her to put in physician mailboxes.

Surprisingly little has been written on patient perceptions of their physicians receiving gifts from the PI, despite the very public nature of this topic and potential consequences for patient care. Mainous et al. surveyed 649 adults in Kentucky in 1994 [1]. Eighty-two percent of individuals surveyed were aware that physicians received gifts with a possible patient benefit, for example, medication samples, pens and pads of paper. In contrast, only 32% of respondents were aware that physicians received personal gifts, such as dinner at an expensive restaurant, clocks or radios [1].

Blake and Early surveyed 486 adults in a family practice outpatient setting in Missouri in 1994. Again, almost 80% of patients were not aware of many gifts commonly provided to doctors, such as meals. Also, respondents distinguished between types of gifts; approval ratings were high for gifts considered to be trivial or having value to patient care [2].

Gibbons et al. compared attitudes of 268 physicians with those of 196 patients toward pharmaceutical industry gifts. Participants were asked to rate 10 pharmaceutical gifts on whether they were likely to influence prescribing. The list included drug samples, a pen, a clock, and so on. About 54% of respondents were aware of such gifts, and of those who had been unaware, 24% responded that this knowledge altered their perception of the medical profession. This subset was found to rate gifts as less appropriate and more influential on prescribing practices. Hence, it is likely that their perception of the medical profession was altered in a negative way. When patients were asked whether they thought their own physician accepted gifts, 27% said yes, 20% said no and 53% were unsure. Furthermore, patient–physician differences concerning the influence of gifts were present even for gifts that existing guidelines consider acceptable, such as meals, pens and textbooks [3].

In all three studies, patients with at least a high school education were significantly likely to believe that personal gifts have a negative effect on the cost of health care [1–3].

Jane finished the chart documentation on her previous patient. She enjoyed her elective at the mental health services clinic, as she had a particular interest in the psychiatric issues of her patients. Her next patient was a middle-aged married woman who had been seeing Jane for treatment of depression after her husband had become ill with cancer. Jane liked this patient, who was bright and engaging, but the initial treatment phase had been notable for significant resistance to seeking help for her symptoms. The patient had many concerns about the "stigma" of mental illness. Jane was proud of the work she had done in help-ing to cultivate trust between herself and the patient, and they had successfully overcome this initial hurdle; the patient came for weekly cognitive behavioral therapy and was now improving significantly. Jane was surprised, then, when her patient came in to her office appearing upset and annoyed. Apparently, while waiting in the clinic for her appointment, she had overheard a pharmaceutical company representative talking to the recep-tionist. He was talking about a free lunch he had arranged for doctors at Zucci's, one of the most expensive restaurants in town. Jane's patient had often talked about the financial diffi-culties her family was facing because of her husband's bills and the cost of his medicines. "It upsets me that drug companies spend so much on freebies to doctors. Have you ever accepted one of these free meals?" Jane's patient asked her.

Types of Gifts

Small Items

Among patients interviewed in these studies, there was a much higher awareness of gifts to doctors such as pens or drug samples. A pen that exhibits the name of a drug is almost certainly more identifiable as a gift from a pharmaceutical company than a book or dinner [1, 2].

Furthermore patients seemed less likely to object to trivial gifts such as pens than to gifts that had some monetary value and offered no clear benefits to patients. Still, receipts of gifts that may be perceived as innocuous, such as pens and pads of paper, were perceived by more than a quarter of patients as having a negative effect on the cost of health care [1].

Medication Samples

Of one sample of patients, 75% reported receiving free samples from their physicians [1]. Eighty-seven percent of another population was aware that physicians received free drug samples from the pharmaceutical industry. Only 7.6% of this sample disapproved of medication samples in the form of gifts [2]. Interestingly, patients in one study who had received medication samples were more likely than nonexposed respondents to view personal gifts as having a negative effect on the cost of health care. They were also less likely to believe that personal gifts had a positive effect on health care quality. The authors speculated that this may be because they were more aware of personal contact between the drug industry and physicians and thus were more concerned that personal gifts to physicians could influence prescribing behaviors [1].

Meals and Hospitality

The PI frequently funds meals at conferences in hospitals or medical offices, yet only 24% of patients surveyed were aware of this practice. Forty-seven percent of the sample reported that "it was not all right" for physicians to accept a gift in the form of dinner at a restaurant [2].

Continuing Medical Education and Conferences

In one study, 32.5% of patients did not approve of their physicians accepting payment by a pharmaceutical company of medical conference expenses and more than 30% disapproved of their physicians attending social events sponsored by pharmaceutical companies at a medical conference [2].

Summary

☐ Patients are often unaware of many personal gifts that are frequently given to physicians by the PI.

☐ When made aware, a significant percentage of patients disapprove of gifts that do not directly benefit patient care.

☐ Patients tend to find gifts from the PI less appropriate than do physicians.

☐ Patients are more likely than physicians to believe acceptance of pharmaceutical gifts may influence prescribing behaviors.

References

1. Mainous AG 3rd, Hueston WJ, Rich EC. Patient perceptions of physician acceptance of gifts from the pharmaceutical industry. Arch Fam Med 1995; 4(4):335–9

2. Blake RL Jr., Early EK. Patients' attitudes about gifts to physicians from pharmaceutical companies. J Am Board Fam Pract 1995; 8(6):457–64

3. Gibbons, RV, Landry FJ, Blouch DL, Jones DL, Williams FK, Lucey CR, Kroenke K. A comparison of physicians' and patients' attitudes toward pharmaceutical industry gifts. J Gen Intern Med 1998; 13(3): 151–4

9 To Sample or Not to Sample? The Use of Pharmaceutical Industry– Supplied Medications in Medical Practice

Bob had just received a call from the clinic nurse, Pat, at the local county family practice clinic. She had requested more samples of Vivre, as the clinic supplies were running low. Bob was pleased that Vivre was being prescribed. Having a presence in the sample closets of local medical clinics was a good way of introducing the medication to prescribers. It also helped to dislodge the current antidepressant market leader from its entrenched position. In addition, MedCorp had launched a direct-to-consumer advertising campaign that was building demand among patients coming into their doctors' offices. Bob told the nurse he would stop by to drop off more samples later that afternoon.

Free medication samples are frequently used by medical clinics [1, 2]. The pharmaceutical industry provides free samples to physicians to promote the use of their products, with market analyses showing that sampling increases drug sales [3–8]. Industry spent a total of $7.9 billion on drug sampling in the year 2000 in the United States [9]. Despite this, issues surrounding the use of samples are often not addressed in medical training. Residents in training are often unaware of important institutional policies regarding sampling, and only 50% of one group felt that they had received adequate training on these issues in medical school [2]. Researchers have reported that among trainees who use samples for their patients, poor prescribing habits often result [4, 5, 8–11]. The need to better educate health professional trainees on the pros and cons of sampling has also been highlighted [2, 3, 5].

The clinic nurse, Pat, asked Jane to sign for the samples that the Vivre rep had arrived with. Jane gladly agreed, and Pat showed Bob into her office. Jane was always grateful for samples. The patients she saw at the county clinic had very limited financial resources. Finding low-cost sources of medication for some of them was always an uphill battle and very frustrating. With county budget cuts there was limited manpower allocated to finding medications, and Jane always resented spending her valuable patient time on this. Samples from the reps were an easy way of getting medications to patients. Jane thanked Bob as she signed for the samples. Bob chatted about the results of a new study indicating that Vivre had fewer sexual side effects than other antidepressants. Bob suggested that Jane use it for her patients for whom this might be an undesirable consequence of antidepressant therapy. He offered her an article, which she accepted and placed on her ever-growing "to read" pile in the corner of her office.

The Advantages of Using Medication Samples

☐ Medication samples are a way of providing free medication to financially needy patients [4, 6, 12–14].
☐ Their use can promote patient goodwill [15].
☐ Sampling provides a way of evaluating the effectiveness and tolerability of the medication for a patient before they invest in a prescription [4, 6, 13, 14].
☐ Physicians (for example, dermatologists) can demonstrate the use of expensive topical agents to their patients so they do not waste the medication [8].

☐ Medication samples can provide immediate relief to patients in distress and can eliminate a trip to the pharmacy [3, 6, 13].

☐ Meeting with pharmaceutical company representatives providing the samples gives the clinician the opportunity to learn about new formulations, new dosages and drug combinations.

Jane's next patient was new to her. The patient was a 23-year-old man who was single and currently employed in a sales job. He gave a classic history of major depressive episodes since the age of 18 for which he had received no treatment, particularly pharmacological therapies. Sadly his untreated depression had contributed to the loss of his job as a computer analyst, and he was currently employed as a retail clerk. His major resistance to seeking pharmacological treatment was a fear of the side effects of medication, particularly sexual side effects. He was finally in a long-term relationship and did not want to jeopardize this in any way. Given his lack of health insurance, Jane gave him a 60-day supply of Vivre in the form of samples, emphasizing its low sexual side effects profile. When she saw the patient 8 weeks later, he reported considerable improvement in his mood and other depressive symptoms. In fact, he had gotten a promotion at work with health benefits as part of the package. Given his change of insurance status, Jane gave him a written prescription for Vivre with a follow-up appointment for 3 months. The patient called the clinic a few hours later. Apparently his insurance provided limited prescription coverage and he was simply unable to afford the monthly copay. Jane was surprised to hear what a 1-month supply of Vivre actually cost and checked with the local pharmacy as to the cost of other medications in the same class. She was astounded by how inexpensive some of them were in comparison. She spent a few minutes critically reviewing the glossy reprint of the article on the side effects profile of Vivre and was disappointed to find some methodological flaws that undermined the conclusions. Jane wondered if she had been hasty in prescribing this new medication when an older, cheaper medication might have been equally effective.

The Disadvantages of Using Medication Samples

☐ Patients receiving medication samples often do not receive the benefit of pharmacy counseling; instructions accompanying the dispensing of samples are often only verbal, and it is hard to track or identify potential drug–drug interactions [2, 4, 13, 15].

☐ Often clinicians who dispense medications neglect to label them with dose and quantity, and this has additional legal implications [2, 13].

☐ Many clinics display very little structure in the organization and dispensing of samples. Lack of documentation makes effective recall of defective medications impossible [13].

☐ Sample medications are usually the most expensive of several options [2, 5, 6, 16]. When these free samples are gone or unavailable, patients are left to pay for these drugs on their own at a cost much higher than generics in the same class.

☐ There is waste in the form of unused sample medications that expire [6].

☐ Identifying which patients have no alternative means of paying for medication is often not easy for health care workers or understood by patients [1, 17].

☐ The use of "free" medication prevents physicians and staff from appreciating the costs of medications [5, 8]; patients have learned to expect samples from their visits to doctor's offices and frequently ask for them [2, 6].

☐ The waste generated by the unique packing of medication samples in the United States alone has been calculated to be 5140 metric tons per year [18].

☐ Historically, samples have been fraudulently diverted for sale [9, 14].

☐ Other safety concerns have been the personal use of medication samples by physicians, office staff and pharmaceutical company representatives [2, 5, 9, 13, 19].

Medication Samples as Gifts to Physicians from the Pharmaceutical Industry

Medication samples can be seen as a gift to physicians from the pharmaceutical industry. Physicians accepting samples of a new drug have shown increased awareness of and preference for the drug [20]. If physicians make personal use of the samples, the effect could be more powerful, with unsuspected and undesirable influences on prescribing behavior [5, 8, 11, 17]. Although personal use of samples by physicians is seen as acceptable, the risk involved in being one's own physician has also been well recognized.

Summary

☐ Medication sampling is common in medical practice.

☐ The availability of samples is useful and often crucial in providing much-needed medications to financially disadvantaged patients.

☐ Medication sampling is also a method used by industry to promote sales.

☐ The advantages and disadvantages of using sample medications should be weighed carefully before deciding what medication to prescribe for a patient at any given time.

☐ Physicians in training are often unaware of important institutional policies surrounding sampling and often feel they receive inadequate training on this issue.

References

1. Wolf BL. Drug samples: Benefit or bait? JAMA 1998; 279(21): 1698–9

2. Shaughnessy AF, Bucci KK. Drug samples and family practice residents. Ann Pharmacother 1997; 31(11):1296–300

3. Groves KE, Sketris I, Tett SE. Prescription drug samples – does this marketing strategy counteract policies for quality use of medications? J Clin Pharm Ther 2003; 28(4):259–71

4. Chew LD, O'Young TS, Hazlet TK, Bradley KA, Maynard C, Lessler DS. A physicians survey of the effect of drug sample availability on physicians' behavior. J Gen Intern Med 2000; 15(7):478–83

5. Westfall JM, McCabe J, Nicholas RA. Personal use of drug samples by physician and office staff. JAMA 1997; 278(2):141–3

6. Coolidge MP. Drug samples: Friend or foe? J Drugs Dermatol 2002; 1(1):49–52

7. Rosenthal MB, Berndt ER, Donahue JM, Frank RG, Epstein AM. Promotion of prescription drugs to consumers. N Engl J Med 2002; 346(7):498–505

8. Storrs FJ. Drug samples: A conflict of interest? Arch Dermatol 1988; 124(8):1283–5

9. Morelli D, Koenigsberg MR. Sample medication dispensing in a residency practice. J Fam Pract 1992; 34(1):42–8

10. Westfall JM, McCabe J, Nicholas RA. Personal use of drug samples by physicians and office staff, author reply. JAMA 1997; 278(19): 1568–9

11. O'Young T, Hazlet TK. Removal of drug samples from two teaching institutions. Am J Health Syst Pharm 2000; 57(12):1179–80

12. Mehta HJ. Personal use of drug samples by physicians and office staff. JAMA 1997; 278(19):1568

13. Backer El, Lebsack JA, Van Tonder RJ, Crabtree BF. The value of pharmaceutical representative visits and medication samples in community-based family practices. J Fam Pract 2000; 49(9):811–16

14. Weary PE. Free drug samples, use and abuse. Arch Dermatol 1988; 124(1):135–7

15. Lurk JT, DeJong DJ, Woods TM, Knell ME, Carroll CA. Effect of changes in patient cost sharing and drug sample policies on prescription drug costs and utilization in a safety net–provider setting. Am J Health Syst Pharm 2004; 61(3):267–72

16. Haxby DG, Rodriguez GS, Zechnich AD, Schuff RA, Tanigawa JS. Manufacturers' distribution of drug samples to a family medicine clinic. Am J Health Syst Pharm 1995; 52(5):496–9

17. Weiner S, Dischler J, Horvitz C. Beyond pharmaceutical manufacturer assistance: Broadening the scope of an indigent drug program. Am J Health Syst Pharm 2001; 58(2):146–50

18. Paj MP, Gracie DM., Bertino JS Jr. Waste generation of drug product samples versus prescriptions obtained through pharmacy dispensing. Pharmacotherapy 2000; 20(5):593–5

19. Tong KL, Lien CY. Do pharmaceutical representatives misuse their drug samples? Can Fam Physician 1995; 41:1363–6

20. Wazana A. Physicians and the pharmaceutical industry. Is a gift ever just a gift? JAMA 2000; 283(3):373–80

10 Physician–Pharmaceutical Industry Interactions (PPIIs), the Law and the Media

Jack left the faculty meeting and headed to clinic. He was not looking forward to his next patient, Mrs. Allison. She was a middle-aged woman with poorly controlled hypertension and Type II diabetes. She had been seen by a string of physicians before him and tried on several different medications. She always left Jack feeling a little frustrated, as she spent more than the allotted appointment time complaining about medication side effects and how "no one was helping her," yet she had questionable compliance with her medication regime and had not lost weight as he had strongly recommended many months ago.

The debate about the nature of the relationship between the medical profession and the pharmaceutical industry (PI) is a very public one. The negative aspects of the relationship have come under intense criticism in major national newspapers. Such articles have originated from a variety of sources, from medical school faculty [1, 2] as well as journalists. Faculty have publicly highlighted concerns over the influence of PI on medical trainees' prescribing behavior [1], as well as over the influence of PI on physicians through industry sponsorship of CME, free gifts and food [2].

With the PI consistently topping the list of the most profitable industries in the United States [3], its practices have come under much scrutiny in the past several years. Drug companies are being publicly targeted in legal cases over such issues as suppressing negative data from clinical trials [4]; illegal marketing activities to physicians [5, 6]; and patient privacy violations [7].

The specific relationship of gift giving from the PI to physicians to try to persuade doctors to prescribe particular pills has been publicized in detail in the mainstream media [8]: "They (drug makers) once routinely offered free dinners, gasoline and even Christmas trees to doctors willing to listen to their sales pitches."

The susceptibility of physicians to industry-supplied "corrupted information" and its consequences for patient care were publicly analyzed in the case against Pfizer, who paid $420 million in fines after pleading guilty to paying doctors to prescribe its epilepsy drug Neurontin [5]. (The illegal marketing was conducted by Warner-Lambert before Pfizer acquired that company in 2000.) The reliance of the PI on doctors to "sell" their drugs has also been highlighted in national newspapers with a detailed account of how a speaker is hired, the return on investment by the drug company for hiring physician speakers and the average speaker honorarium [9].

Mrs. Allison listed her complaints about the current medication, and Jack wondered what to do. He did not think she was taking the medication as prescribed, and she did not appear to want to take responsibility for her own care. He felt confused and frustrated and uncomfortable. He prided himself on his confidence in his decisions about patient management. He decided to take the patient off her current antihypertensive and put her on Lowpress. As he discussed the risks and benefits of the medication, she started to shake her head and said mockingly, "You doctors all have your favorites, don't you?" She pointed to the pen Jack was using to write the script, which was emblazoned with the "Lowpress" logo. (He had just picked it up at the faculty meeting where Brown Pharmaceuticals had sponsored lunch.)

Jack ignored her comments and continued with his advice, handed her the script and showed her out of the office. Afterward he sat down and found himself feeling very angry. "How dare she question my integrity!" he thought. "Just because I use their pen and eat their lunch does not mean I am influenced by them." He continued with the rest of his clinic feeling indignant.

The Law and PPII

Government regulators have been increasingly interested in PPII. (For resultant policies and codes of conduct, please refer to Chapter 7.) Physician gifts from pharmaceutical company representatives may invoke antikickback laws; both physicians and the pharmaceutical companies are vulnerable, with the possibility of criminal prosecution, civil monetary fines and exclusion from government programs [10, 11].

PPII and Antikickback Laws

If a physician receives such a gift, financial or otherwise, from a pharmaceutical company in exchange for prescribing a drug,[1] federal antikickback laws can be invoked. Prosecutors have begun to apply the antikickback laws to cases dealing with interactions between physicians and the pharmaceutical companies. This is illustrated in the case of TAP Pharmaceuticals and Lupron, a potent gonadotropin-releasing hormone agonist used in the treatment of prostate cancer. Practices such as trips to resorts, consulting arrangements with no work product and open-ended educational grants came under scrutiny, and eventually TAP entered into a settlement with the government in which it agreed to pay $290 million in criminal fines plus $585 million in civil penalties [12].

---

[1] If the drug is reimbursable under Medicare, Medicaid or other government-sponsored health insurance program.

Physician–Drug Company Relationship: Permissible and Impermissible Conduct and Ethical Considerations

Impermissible Conduct	Permissible Conduct
Receiving gifts such as sporting event tickets, spa visits, lavish dinners, or golf outings from drug companies.	Receiving most meals or other gifts that serve an educational function.
Receiving a direct payment or subsidy to attend a continuing education seminar. This includes travel cost, lodging, or other personal costs.	Receiving textbooks that serve an educational function.
Receiving cash payments from a drug company or other things of value in relation to the physician's prescribing practices.	Receiving gifts such as pens or notepads if related to the physician's work. Educational and practice-related items must be for the benefit of the patients and worth less than $100 per item.
Being retained as a sham "consultant" as a reward for prescribing the company's drug.	Legitimate consultation and research (trial program) retainers are allowed if the physician has particular expertise and such expertise is valuable to the clinical trial.
Compensation for the time attending a conference or lavish meals or social events as part of the conference.	Receiving free hospitality or modest social events if part of a conference.

(continued)

55

Impermissible Conduct	Permissible Conduct
Requesting that a drug company furnish free drugs for personal or family use or receiving free drugs for long-term treatment of personal or family chronic illness.	Speakers or faculty at conferences may receive reasonable honoraria and travel expenses.
Participating in a raffle whose winners receive a paid vacation from the drug company.	Receipt of drug samples for personal or family use if they do not interfere with patient access to drug samples.

Table taken from Beatty Y. Gifts from pharmaceutical reps: Exercise caution. Tenn Med 2005; 98(1). Reprinted with the permission of Tennessee Medical Association and Tennessee Medicine © 2005.

In June 2002, Vermont became the first state to require pharmaceutical companies to file annual reports disclosing gifts or payment to physicians exceeding a certain value [13].

Since the implementation of guidelines (refer to Chapter 7), a range of activities that had previously been ubiquitous, for example, receiving gifts such as sporting event tickets or cruises or being paid directly to attend conferences, are now seen as unethical and even illegal. This said, the extent of compliance with voluntary industry and medicine society guidelines remains unknown.

Another area under increasing public and legal scrutiny is physician researchers working with the PI; issues such as gag clauses in clinical trial agreements and failure to disclose information that physicians are duty-bound to disclose make both the physician and the PI liable [14].

Summary

☐ The debate about the nature of the relationship between the medical professional and the pharmaceutical industry is a public one.

☐ Government regulators have been increasingly interested in PPII.

☐ Physicians must be aware of permissible and impermissible conduct with drug companies.

References

1. Shapiro D. Drug companies get too close for medical school's comfort. http://query.nytimes.com/gst/fullpage.html?res=9F00E2D81439F933A15752C0A9629C8B63&sec=health&pagewanted=2 Last accessed 12/2006

2. Relman AS. Your doctor's drug problem. http://www.dearshrink.com/nytimes_docsdrugprob111803.pdf. Last accessed 12/2006

3. Napoli M. Drug industry most profitable. Health Facts 2002; 27(5):31/4P

4. Wadman M. Spitzer sues drug giant for deceiving doctors. Nature 2004; 429(10):589

5. Harris G. Pfizer to pay $420 million in illegal marketing case. The New York Times. May 14, 2004. Page C6

6. Kowalcyzk L. Pfizer unit agrees to $430 million in fines. Boston Globe. May 14, 2001. Page D1

7. Yamey G. Eli Lilly violates patients' privacy. BMJ 2001; 323(7304):65

8. Harris G. Drug makers are still giving gifts to doctors, FDA officials tell senators. The New York Times. March 4, 2005. Page A15

9. Hensley S, Martinez B. To sell their drugs, companies increasingly rely on doctors. Wall Street Journal. July 15, 2005. Pages A1, A2

10. Beatty Y. Gifts from pharmaceutical representatives: Exercise caution. Tenn Med 2005; 981(1):33–4

11. Robinson DJ. Interactions between drug reps and physicians. Physicians News Digest 2004 (April):1–3

12. Studdert DM, Mello MM, Brennan TA. Financial conflicts of interest in physicians' relationships with the pharmaceutical industry – self regulation in the shadow of federal prosecution. N Engl J Med 2004; 351(18):1891–900

13. Tsai AC. Policies to regulate gifts to physicians from the industry. JAMA 2003; 290(13):1776

14. Litman M, Sheremeta L. The report of the Committee of Inquiry on the case involving Dr. Nancy Olivieri: A fiduciary law perspective. Health Law Rev 2002; 10(2):3–13

11 Direct-to-Consumer Advertising (DTCA)

Direct-to-consumer advertising (DTCA)[1] has become one of the most contentious issues facing the medical profession in the United States [1–3]. Before the 1980's, companies marketed their prescription products exclusively to physicians [1, 4]. Since then, with the proliferation of drug formularies, utilization review systems and pharmaceutical risk sharing agreements, physician authority to prescribe specific drugs has been eroded and companies have turned marketing efforts to consumers [5]. Only the United States and New Zealand allow advertising of prescription drugs directly to patients [6]. Spending on DTCA of prescription drugs in the United States totaled $3.2 billion in 2003 [7]. Advertising can be found in magazines, on television and on the radio. DTCA in the United States is regulated by the FDA, which examines the commercials after they become available to the public [4].

---

[1] DTCA: promotional efforts by a pharmaceutical company to present prescription drugs or drug therapy information to the general public through the lay media.

Advantages of DTCA

☐ Industry advertising can alert patients to possible diagnoses, risks and potential treatments [8, 10–12].

☐ Better-informed patients comply better with long-term treatment [8].

☐ Industry advertising is controlled through legal and regulatory agency initiatives, in contrast to with other sources of health information such as the Internet. Hence, industry advertising can provide balanced and accurate information to patients [8].

☐ Industry advertising encourages informed communication between patients and providers [1, 10].

☐ Industry advertising encourages patient autonomy; patients are better able to weigh the benefits and risks of their health choices [1, 3, 9, 12].

☐ Ads that appeal to a broad audience and include celebrity endorsements may help reduce the stigma associated with mental illness [9, 12].

Disadvantages of DTCA

☐ People with certain conditions, such as mental illnesses, are more susceptible to being manipulated by promotional efforts [13].

☐ Ads do not fairly convey risks and benefits of the drug [1, 3, 9, 12, 14].

☐ Patient misperception of drugs effectiveness could lead to patient pressure to prescribe inappropriate drugs [12, 14].

☐ Patient misperception of DTCA could lead to patient pressure to prescribe drugs that have no significant benefit over similar medications that are older and also cheaper [3, 12, 14].

□ DTCA can medicalize normal human experience [3, 9, 14]; that is, it can lead people to seek treatments that they do not need.

□ Advertising campaigns cast too wide a net, targeting relatively healthy people because of the need for adequate returns on costly ad campaigns [14].

□ Regulation by the FDA has limitations: Millions of patients can be exposed to misleading ads before regulatory action is taken [3, 9].

□ Financial conflicts of interest taint the information consumers and potential and actual patients receive via DTCA [9].

□ Physicians complain that they must devote increasing amounts of scarce time to dissuading patients from taking drugs that advertising has led them to believe are unproblematic [1].

□ DTCA rarely mentions lifestyle changes or other nonpharmacological interventions, which are often as important as drug therapy in improving outcomes [5].

DTCA and Its Impact on the Physician–Patient Relationship

Studies examining the relationships among DTCA, patients' requests for prescriptions and prescription decisions reveal that patient requests for medicines are a powerful driver of prescribing decisions [6]. Furthermore, although physicians prescribed the requested medicine, they were often ambivalent regarding the choice of medicine. In one study, 39% of physicians perceived DTCA as damaging to the time efficiency of the patient visit; 13% saw it as helpful [11]. A total of 33% of physicians thought that discussing DTCA had improved the doctor–patient relationship; 8% felt it had worsened it. Other studies have replicated these results, with physicians believing that DTCA affected interactions with patients negatively by lengthening clinical encounters [10, 15]. Studies exploring the effect of patients' DTCA-related requests on physicians' initial treatment of patients with depressive symptoms highlighted the competing effects on quality, potentially both averting underuse and promoting overuse [2].

Furthermore, benefits of DTCA might be maximized and harm minimized by increasing the accuracy of information in advertisements, enhancing physicians' communication and negotiation skills and encouraging patients to respect physicians' clinical expertise [11]. Kravitz emphasizes that physicians should meet patient requests with questions: Where did you hear about that drug? What did the ad say? How and where do you hope it would help? What do you know of the drug's benefits and side effects? Tell me more about your symptoms. Would you like to hear more about this drug and its alternates [5]?

Summary

- ☐ DTCA has become one of the most contentious issues facing the medical profession in the United States.
- ☐ Physicians need to be aware of the advantages and disadvantages of DTCA and its potential impact on their relationship with their patients.
- ☐ Physicians should be prepared to meet patients' requests for DTCA medications with appropriate questions.

References

1. Huang AJ. The rise of direct to consumer advertising of prescription drugs in the United States. MSJAMA 2000; 284(17):2240

2. Kravitz RL, Epstein RM, Feldman MD, Franz CE, Azari R, Wilkes MS, Hinton L, Franks P. Influence of patients' requests for direct to consumer advertised antidepressants. A randomized controlled trial. JAMA 2005; 293(16):1995–2002

3. Hollon MF. Direct to consumer advertising: A haphazard approach to health promotion. JAMA 2005; 293(16):2030–3

4. Henney JE. Challenges in regulating direct to consumer advertising. JAMA 2000; 284(17):2242

5. Kravitz RL. Direct to consumer advertising of prescription drugs: Implications for the patient-physician relationship. MSJAMA 2000; 284(17):2244

6. Mintzes B, Barer ML, Kravitz RL, Kazanjian A, Bassett K, Lexchin J, Evans RG, Pan R, Marion SA. Influence of direct to consumer pharmaceutical advertising and patients' requests on prescribing decisions: 2 site cross sectional survey. BMJ 2002; 324(7332):278–9

7. IMS Health. Jan 2000–Dec 2000. Prescription drug trends. Fact Sheet 3057–03. Kaiser Family Foundation, Menlo Park, CA, 2004

8. Bonaccorso SN, Sturchio JL. For and against: Direct to consumer advertising is medicalizing normal human experience: Against. BMJ 2002; 324(7342):910–11

9. Lenhardt E. Why so glum? Toward a fair balance of competitive interests in direct to consumer advertising and the well being of the mentally ill consumers it targets. Health Matrix Cleveland 2005; 15(1):165–204

10. Robinson AR, Hohmann KB, Rifkin J, Topp D, Gilroy CM, Pickard JA, Anderson RJ. Direct to consumer pharmaceutical advertising. Arch Intern Med 2004; 164(4):427–32

11. Murray E, Lo B, Pollack L, Donelar K, Lee K. Direct-to-consumer advertising: Physician views of its effects on quality of care and the doctor-patient relationship. J Am Board Fam Pract 2003; 16(6):513–24

12. Chin MH. The patient's role in choice of medications: Direct to consumer advertising and patient decision aids. Yale J Health Policy Law Ethics 2005; 5(2):771–84

13. Freudenheim M. Psychiatric drugs are now promoted directly to patients. http://query.nytimes.com/gst/fullpage.html?sec=health&res =9503E6D8163FF934A25751C0A96E958260 Last accessed 12/2006

14. Mintzes B. For and against: Direct to consumer advertising is medicalizing normal human experience: For. BMJ 2002; 324(7342): 908–9

15. Maubach N, Hoek J. New Zealand general practitioners' views on direct-to-consumer advertising of prescription medicines: A qualitative analysis. N Z Med J 2005; 118(1215):U1543

12

Pharmaceutical Industry Interactions with Health Care Professionals

A Global Perspective

The debate over physician–pharmaceutical industry interactions (PPIIs) is clearly a global one. The World Health Organization has published "criteria for medicinal drug promotion and the code of pharmaceutical marketing practice" for countries without national codes [1]. The World Medical Association also published guidelines in 2004 [2]. The ethical and legal conflicts of PPII have been highlighted in the medical literature from Norway [3, 4], Poland [5], Germany [6, 7], Australia [8–10], Spain [11], India [12, 13], Sri Lanka [14] and Turkey [15].

The pharmaceutical industry interacts not only with physicians but also with other health care professionals such as nurses, nurse practitioners and physician assistants; with health care organizations such as HMOs; and with consumer organizations and pharmacists.

Pharmaceutical companies and patient organizations frequently come together to explore areas of shared interest [16]. Some have argued that these offer the PI a chance to mobilize grassroots lobbying muscle to influence policymakers [17]. Serious issues have recently been highlighted concerning undeclared interests in commercial funding of charitable and lay organizations without apparent conflict [18].

In addition, the PI relationship with HMOs, including rebate policies, formulary decision making, intervention activities, disease management programs and Medicaid rebate calculations, has recently come under federal scrutiny [19].

In Canada, potential patient identifiers and physician-linked prescription data stream from pharmacy computers via commercial compliers to pharmaceutical companies without the informed consent of patients and physicians [20]. Buying prescriber data provides pharmaceutical sales representatives the ability to precisely target their promotional efforts to react to changes in prescribing behavior [21].

Nurses are also the recipients of gifts from the PI, and nursing as a profession has recognized the practice as a growing threat to nursing integrity. However, there is a gap in the literature regarding actual PI influence on nurse practitioner prescribing patterns [23] despite frequent interactions in the form of free food, sponsorship of CME and medication samples [24, 25].

References

1. Wager E. How to dance with porcupines: Rules and guidelines on doctors' relations with drug companies. BMJ 2003; 326(7400):1196–8

2. Kmietowicz Z. WMA sets rules on how doctors handle industry sponsorship. BMJ 2004; 329(7471):876

3. Aasland OG, Forde R. Physicians and drug industry: Attitudes and practice. Tidiskrift for Den Norske Laegeforening 2004; 124(20): 2603–6

4. Haug C. Dangerously tempting fellowships. Tidiskrift for Den Norske Laegeforening 2004; 124(20):2597

5. Zimmerman R, Romanowski M, Malach P. The legal evaluation of contacts between a physician and a pharmacological company. Klin Oczna 2004; 106(6):809–11

6. Haser I, Hofmann A. New conduct recommendations for physicians cooperating with the pharmaceutical industry? The "FS Codex" and its consequences for physicians. Anaesthesist 2005; 54(3):263–7

7. Helmchen H. Psychiatrists and the pharmaceutical industry. Nervenarzt 2003; 74(11):955–64

8. Komesaroff PA. Ethical issues in the relationships with industry: An ongoing challenge. J Pediatr Child Health 2005; 41(11):558–60

9. Henry DA, Kerridge IH, Hill SR, McNeill PM, Doran E, Newby DA, Henderson KM, Maguire J, Stokes BJ, MacDonald GJ, Day RO. Medical specialists and the pharmaceutical industry sponsored research: A survey of the Australian experience. Med J Aust 2005; 182 (11):557–60

10. Komesaroff PA, Kerridge IH. Ethical issues concerning the relationships between medical practitioners and the pharmaceutical industry. Med J Aust 2002; 176(3):118–21

11. Estevez De Vidts A. Physicians and the hospitality of pharmaceutical companies. Rev Med Chil 2004; 132(4):522

12. Ravindran GD. The physician and the pharmaceutical industry: Both must keep the patient's interests at heart. Issues Med Ethics 1999; 7(1):21–2

13. Bal A. Can the medical profession and the pharmaceutical industry work ethically for better health care? Indian J Med Ethics 2004; 1(1):17

14. Malavige GN. Doctors, drug companies and medical ethics: A Sri Lankan perspective. Indian J Med Ethics 2004; 1(1):26

15. Tengilimoglu D, Kisa A, Ekiyor A. The pharmaceutical sales rep/physician relationship in Turkey: Ethical issues in an international context. Health Mark Q 2004; 22(1):21–39

16. Herxheimer A. Relationships between the pharmaceutical industry and patients organization. BMJ 2003; 326(7400):1208–10

17. Burton B, Rowell A. An unhealthy spin. BMJ 2003; 326(7400):1205–7

18. Hirst J. Charities and patient groups should declare interests. BMJ 2003; 326(7400):1211

19. Benko LB. Managed care gets a closer look from feds. Mod Health 2002; 32(21):10–11

20. Zoutman DE, Ford BD, Bassili AR. The confidentiality of patient and physician information in pharmacy prescription records. CMAJ 2004; 170(5):815–16

21. Pearson LJ, Can prescriber profiling happen to you? Nurse Pract 2003; 28(12):8

22. Stokamer CL. Pharmaceutical gift giving: Analysis of an ethical dilemma. J Nurs Adm 2003; 33(1):48–51

23. Sidiqi S, Edmund M. Pharmaceutical influence? Nurse Pract 2003; 28(5):6–7

24. Gerchufsky M. Decoding the sales pitch. Adv Nurse Pract 1997; 5(6):65–6

25. Edmunds M. Who's supporting your CE program? Nurse Pract 2002; 27(7):47

13 Internet Resources for Teaching about PPII and Independent Sources of Information about Prescription Medicines

There are many helpful Internet resources for teaching physicians about PPII. No Free Lunch (http://www.nofreelunch.org, last accessed June 2006) is a website run by health care providers who believe that "pharmaceutical promotion should not guide clinical practice and that over zealous promotional practices can lead to bad patient care." It receives no external funding.

The impetus for the World Health Organization (WHO)/Non-Governmental Organizations (NGO) Drug Promotion Database started in May 1999 at the WHO/Public Interest NGO Roundtable on Pharmaceuticals. This website (www.drugpromo.info, last accessed June 2006) is coordinated by WHO's Department of Essential Drugs and Medicines Policy and Health Action International Europe. It has input from health care professionals globally. The website systematically documents evidence for various types of pharmaceutical promotion on physicians and critically reviews the research in this area.

The American Medical Association's *AMA Virtual Mentor* is the online ethics and professionalism journal of the AMA. Its mission is to "promote the ethical and professional development of tomorrow's physicians." In July 2003 it published an issue on medicine and industry that can be accessed at www.ama-assn.org/ama/pub/category/10812.html (last accessed June 2006).

The American Medical Students Association (AMSA) Pharm-Free campaign started in 2002 in collaboration with No Free Lunch (www.amsa.org/prof/pharmfree.cfm, last accessed June 2006) and could be a useful source of discussion for medical student curricula.

The Medical Letter is a nonprofit organization founded in 1958 (www.medicalletter.org, last accessed June 2006). It is completely independent, supported solely by fees, and accepts no advertising, grants or donations.

Prescriber's Letter is totally independent and has no connection with any pharmaceutical firm. There is no advertising or other financial support (http://www.prescribersletter.com/, last accessed June 2006).

Appendix I

About Opinion 8.061, "Gifts to Physicians from Industry"

Over time, many gifts to physicians from pharmaceutical, device and medical equipment industry sales representatives have served an important and beneficial function. For example, industry has provided funds for educational seminars and conferences for many years.

During the late 1980's, however, some of these gifts were becoming lavish, ranging from frequent flier miles to cash and trips to luxury resorts, and their appropriateness was increasingly being called into question. The AMA studied the issue, and in December of 1990, the AMA's House of Delegates adopted CEJA's ethical guidelines to prevent inappropriate gift-giving practices. The AMA's "Guidelines on Gifts to Physicians from Industry" later appeared in its Code of Medical Ethics (CEJA Ethical Opinion 8.061).

The Pharmaceutical Manufacturer's Association (PMA), which later became PhRMA (Pharmaceutical Research and Manufacturers of America), also adopted the guidelines.

Opinion 8.061, "Gifts to Physicians from Industry"

Many gifts given to physicians by companies in the pharmaceutical, device, and medical equipment industries serve an important and socially beneficial function. For example, companies have long provided funds for educational seminars and conferences. However, there has been growing concern about certain gifts from industry to physicians. Some gifts that reflect customary practices of industry may not be consistent with the Principles of Medical Ethics. To avoid the acceptance of inappropriate gifts, physicians should observe the following guidelines:

(1) Any gifts accepted by physicians individually should primarily entail a benefit to patients and should not be of substantial value. Accordingly, textbooks, modest meals, and other gifts are appropriate if they serve a genuine educational function. Cash payments should not be accepted. The use of drug samples for personal or family use is permissible as long as these practices do not interfere with patient access to drug samples. It would not be acceptable for non-retired physicians to request free pharmaceuticals for personal use or use by family members.

(2) Individual gifts of minimal value are permissible as long as the gifts are related to the physician's work (e.g., pens and notepads).

(3) The Council on Ethical and Judicial Affairs defines a legitimate "conference" or "meeting" as any activity, held at an appropriate location, where (a) the gathering is primarily dedicated, in both time and effort, to promoting objective scientific and educational activities and discourse (one or more educational presentation(s) should be the highlight of the gathering), and (b) the main incentive for bringing attendees together is to further their knowledge on the topic(s) being presented. An appropriate disclosure of financial support or conflict of interest should be made.

(4) Subsidies to underwrite the costs of continuing medical education conferences or professional meetings can contribute to the improvement of patient care and therefore are permissible. Since the giving of a subsidy directly to a physician by a company's representative may create a relationship that could influence the use of the company's

products, any subsidy should be accepted by the conference's sponsor who in turn can use the money to reduce the conference's registration fee. Payments to defray the costs of a conference should not be accepted directly from the company by the physicians attending the conference.

(5) Subsidies from industry should not be accepted directly or indirectly to pay for the costs of travel, lodging, or other personal expenses of physicians attending conferences or meetings, nor should subsidies be accepted to compensate for the physicians' time. Subsidies for hospitality should not be accepted outside of modest meals or social events held as a part of a conference or meeting. It is appropriate for faculty at conferences or meetings to accept reasonable honoraria and to accept reimbursement for reasonable travel, lodging, and meal expenses. It is also appropriate for consultants who provide genuine services to receive reasonable compensation and to accept reimbursement for reasonable travel, lodging, and meal expenses. Token consulting or advisory arrangements cannot be used to justify the compensation of physicians for their time or their travel, lodging, and other out-of-pocket expenses.

(6) Scholarship or other special funds to permit medical students, residents, and fellows to attend carefully selected educational conferences may be permissible as long as the selection of students, residents, or fellows who will receive the funds is made by the academic or training institution. Carefully selected educational conferences are generally defined as the major educational, scientific or policy-making meetings of national, regional or specialty medical associations.

(7) No gifts should be accepted if there are strings attached. For example, physicians should not accept gifts if they are given in relation to the physician's prescribing practices. In addition, when companies underwrite medical conferences or lectures other than their own, responsibility for and control over the selection of content, faculty, educational methods, and materials should belong to the organizers

of the conferences or lectures. (II) Issued June 1992 based on the report "Gifts to Physicians from Industry," adopted December 1990 (JAMA. 1991; 265: 501 and Food and Drug Law Journal. 2001; 56: 27–40); Updated June 1996 and June 1998.

In response to frequent questions, an addendum to Opinion E-8.061 is offered for clarification.

Academy of Pharmaceutical Physicians

and Investigators

Code of Ethics for the Practice of

Pharmaceutical Medicine

Preamble

Academy of Pharmaceutical Physicians and Investigators (APPI) Code of Ethics for the Practice of Pharmaceutical Medicine complements the Academy's Mission, Objectives and Purpose [1].

The APPI Code of Ethics sets the standard of conduct and behavior for APPI members responsible for medical considerations in pharmaceutical and medical device research and development, and post-marketing product safety surveillance.

The Code describes the principles that guide ethical decision-making to ensure that the best interests of patients and study participants, as well as their families, doctors, nurses and other health care professionals, are served. The Code seeks to assure safe use of medical products.

The Code establishes a standard for addressing ethical dilemmas in pharmaceutical research and its applications.

The APPI Code of Ethics

Members of the Academy of Pharmaceutical Physicians and Investigators (APPI) accept the fundamental responsibility to:

☐ Give first priority to the well being of participants in research studies and patients who use pharmaceutical products and medical devices.

- ☐ Ensure that potential risks to clinical study participants are minimized, that these risks are fully evaluated against potential benefits, and that potential risks and benefits are clearly communicated to study participants and their physicians.
- ☐ Apply sound ethical values and judgment in the design, conduct and analysis of clinical studies, and in the interpretation of results.
- ☐ Adhere to the principles of good clinical practice and research.
- ☐ Support the dissemination only of scientifically sound information from clinical trials and other investigations, without regard to study outcomes, for the benefit of medicine and science.
- ☐ Ensure that all industry-based, medically relevant product information is fair, balanced, accurate, comprehensive and easily accessible, in order that patients and physicians can make well-informed decisions about the use of pharmaceuticals and medical devices.
- ☐ Strive to understand and respect differences in values across cultures and to appropriately adapt behaviors while maintaining ethical principles.
- ☐ Foster the education and professional competence of AAPP members, to enable them to uphold ethical principles in the practice of pharmaceutical medicine.
- ☐ Appropriately question, consult and advise each other regarding medical and ethical concerns, and to seek external opinions, as appropriate, in the best interests of patients and clinical study participants.

Adopted by the APPI Board of Trustees
14 October 2001
1. MISSION, OBJECTIVES AND PURPOSE OF THE
AMERICAN ACADEMY OF PHARMACEUTICAL
PHYSICIANS, as stated in the BY-LAWS, January 1, 2000

Article II

Section 1. MISSION. To enhance the proficiency of pharmaceutical physicians, the Academy shall promote the acquisition and dissemination of knowledge concerning the therapeutic action, investigation and development of medicines and diagnostics and the protection of the welfare of patients and study subjects.

Section 2. OBJECTIVES AND PURPOSE.

The purposes of the academy shall be to:

Foster the traditional role of the physician as a guardian of health by applying good science and medical judgment to meeting the needs of patients for pharmacotherapeutic uses;

Enhance relationships between pharmaceutical physicians and other members of the medical profession;

Work to enhance the image and professional recognition of pharmaceutical medicine (as defined in Section 12 of Article III) as a specialty;

Assist members in maintaining and enhancing skills and knowledge in pharmaceutical medicine (as defined in Section 12 of Article III);

Function as a nonprofit educational organization of physicians who are in pharmaceutical medicine; and

Provide a forum for the exchange of medical and scientific information pertaining to pharmaceutical medicine.

Principles to Guide the Relationship between Graduate Medical Education and Industry

The Accreditation Council for Graduate Medical Education (ACGME) establishes educational standards for, and monitors compliance by, more than 7,700 residency programs and 700 institutional sponsors of graduate medical education (GME) in the United States. This paper sets forth principles inherent in these standards that address the relationship between GME and industry, with particular emphasis on pharmaceutical companies. The principles outlined herein should guide the efforts of teaching institutions and residency programs to promote reflective and unbiased learning and thus to help form competent professionals who serve the best interests of patients in a consistently ethical and exemplary fashion.

The Problem

A variety of industries have an impact on health care delivery in the United States. These include, but are not limited to, insurers, manufacturers of medical devices, pharmaceutical companies, and developers of educational products and offerings. While each represents a potential source of influence on physician practice, the pharmaceutical industry is decidedly one of the largest and most influential. As reported in 2001, investments in research to discover and identify new medicines by pharmaceutical manufacturers amounted to at least $30.5 billion [1]. Wazana reports that pharmaceuticals' annual promotion and marketing expenditures are estimated to be in excess of $11 billion, with $8,000 to $13,000 of these promotional dollars spent directly or indirectly per year on each physician [2]. While major benefits result from research and development by the pharmaceutical industry, the potential for conflict of interest from promotion and marketing also has been proven [3, 4]. This influence presents a serious threat to the professionalism both of physicians and the institutions that sponsor their educational programs [5, 6].

In their broadest context, the goals of the medical profession and the pharmaceutical industry are aligned around efforts to improve human health through a direct and positive effect on patient care. Benefits to patients result from services provided by both doctors and drug companies. Closer scrutiny, however, of the core relationships maintained by each of these entities reveals an irreconcilable difference. The relationship to its shareholders defines values and influences behaviors held by industry. Thus, for example, the responsibility of the pharmaceutical industry must be to act in the best interests of its shareholders by maximizing their return on investment. In so doing, much good is clearly accomplished for patients. In contrast, however, the altruism expected of medical professionals dictates that doctors put patients first. The doctor-patient relationship, with all its ensuing values, is the foundation of medical professionalism; the good of the patient must be preeminent.

The Challenge for Medical Education

The conflict of values between the professional ethics of the physician and the business ethics of industry is impossible to ignore. Nowhere is this conflict more apparent than in the conduct of promotional activities. Industry engages in advertising campaigns and associated marketing activities because they work; successful promotion increases shareholder value. It is the chief means by which industry relates to physicians, residents, and medical students. Promotion by industry, and pharmaceutical companies in particular, frequently occurs through financial support for a broad array of educational programs, industry-sponsored research, and social events. Many residency programs and clinical departments not only accept but also often actively seek such support, justifying this dependence on the serious budgetary constraints under which they must operate in an increasingly constrained financial environment. Unfortunately, such promotional support has been proven to influence medical decision-making, and studies have found decision makers unable to recognize its impact [7, 8].

Faculty and residents alike communicate professional values through the learning environment created by sponsoring institutions and individual residency programs. The structured curriculum, i.e., conferences, grand rounds, and other formal learning activities, is the most obvious of the contexts in which transmittal of values occurs. While less apparent, though with equal and sometimes even greater intensity, the hidden or informal curriculum communicates values at the level of organizational structure and culture, influencing such areas as policy development, evaluation, resource allocation, and institutional slang [9]. Transmittal of values thus becomes a pervasive component of the educational process relative to all manner of professional relationships within the sponsoring institution and individual training program. Residents learn to relate to industry in much the same manner they develop other professional relationships, by observing individual administration and faculty behavior in the context of the program and sponsoring institution. The learning environment, therefore, has a direct bearing on the "learned" professionalism of the residents training within it [10]. Regrettably, with regard to support from industry, the learning environment often manifests an "entitlement to largesse of drug companies" [5].

Instances of inappropriate relationships with industry and its "largesse" are frequently found in the expectations for outside support demonstrated by residency programs and sponsoring institutions. Examples that have become all-too-familiar practices include: "drug lunches" with obvious promotional intent; industry-sponsored lectures with negative results of clinical trials conveniently given less or no attention; and social functions attached to "information sessions" having a clearer marketing objective than scientific purpose. Recently, concern has arisen over a new variation of a promotional activity in which residents and even medical students receive slides, lecture materials and honoraria and subsequently act as "experts," delivering the packaged information at continuing medical education events. The risk of compromising professional judgment resulting from these and other activities can be egregious, and both the profession and the public continue to express concern over blatant misuse of industry support [11–13].

Existing Guidelines

A number of organizations have developed guidelines for physicians and organizations about accepting gifts and support from industry. Most widely recognized among these guidelines are: the ethical opinion "Gifts to Physicians from Industry" found in the American Medical Association's Code of Medical Ethics [14]; the American College of Physicians–American Society of Internal Medicine position statement on "Physicians and the Pharmaceutical Industry" [15, 16]; "Physicians and the Pharmaceutical Industry" promulgated by the Canadian Medical Association [17]; and, the Accreditation Council for Continuing Medical Education, through its Standards for Commercial Support [18]. The Association of American Medical Colleges (AAMC) has specifically addressed issues regarding financial conflicts of interest in research through the work of its Task Force on Financial Conflicts of Interest in Research [19].

These guidelines outline what constitutes ethical behavior for both physicians and organizations. Without exception, they establish that it is unethical for physicians to accept gifts or support in any form that results in recommendation of a particular product or delivery of particular clinical action. The Standards for Commercial Support [18] regulate use of funds provided by pharmaceutical and other proprietary interests in the sponsorship of continuing medical education events.

The Role of the ACGME

The General Competencies

The ACGME, through its Residency Review and Institutional Review Committees, has identified six general competencies for all physicians in its Program and Institutional Requirements. These competencies—Patient Care, Medical Knowledge, Practice-based Learning and Improvement, Interpersonal and Communication Skills, Professionalism, and Systems-based Practice—serve as organizing principles around which all GME residency curricula should be developed [20]. Residents must demonstrate achievement in these competencies during and upon completion of their residency program through appropriate educational outcomes. The residency program itself must demonstrate improvement based upon the outcomes identified through these assessment activities.

The competencies are not prescriptive rules; they are, however, a conceptual framework for defining program and institutional policies regarding all professional relationships in GME. At present, ACGME standards do not directly address the nature of the professional relationships that exist between residency programs, their sponsoring institutions, and industry. As such, they shed light on behaviors appropriate to the integrity and objectivity that must be maintained within a teaching environment. Using a framework shaped by the general competencies, the principles that follow should guide the conduct of the relationships maintained by residency programs and their sponsoring institutions with industry.

Professionalism

Professionalism is an expression of the norms that guide the relationships in which physicians are engaged [21]. It is, therefore, the competency that stands at the core of how programs and institutions model behavior with regard to relationships with industry. In her review of the literature, Arnold has identified those traits commonly associated with professionalism as altruism, respect for others as embodied in humanistic qualities, honor, integrity, ethical behavior, accountability, excellence, a sense of duty, and advocacy [22]. Ginsburg, et al., have described these traits as context-dependent, that is, demonstrated through behaviors that occur in particular circumstances, often manifesting themselves in conflicts between values [23].

Programmatic and institutional policies must therefore guide action in light of the inherent conflict of values between industry and the medical profession. The following principles promote Professionalism in programs and sponsoring institutions with regard to relationships with industry:

1. Ethics curricula must include instruction in and discussion of published guidelines regarding gift-giving to physicians. Among these guidelines are the ethical opinion "Gifts to Physicians from Industry" found in the Code of Medical Ethics of the American Medical Association [14], the Policy on Physician-Industry Relations of the American College of Physicians–American Society of Internal Medicine [15, 16], "Physicians and the Pharmaceutical Industry" promulgated by the Canadian Medical Association [17], and the ethics statements of various medical specialty societies.
2. Full and appropriate disclosure of sponsorship and financial interests is required at all program and institution-sponsored events, above and beyond those already governed by the

Standards for Commercial Support promulgated by the ACCME [18]. Likewise, full disclosure of research interests must be published in keeping with the local policies of institutional review boards and following the recommendations of the Association of American Medical Colleges (AAMC) Task Force on Financial Conflicts of Interest in Research [19].

3. Programs and sponsoring institutions must determine through policy, which contacts, if any, between residents and industry representatives may be suitable, and exclude occasions in which involvement by industry representatives or promotion of industry products is inappropriate.

Practice-based Learning and Improvement and Medical Knowledge

Practice-Based Learning and Improvement refers to how physicians apply Medical Knowledge by investigating and evaluating their own patient care, appraising and assimilating scientific evidence, and making subsequent improvements in the care of their patients. The following principles informed by Practice-Based Learning and Improvement and Medical Knowledge, apply to the relationship between GME and industry:

1. Clinical skills and judgment must be learned in an objective and evidence-based learning environment.
2. Residents must learn how promotional activities can influence judgment in prescribing decisions and research activities through specific instructional activities.
3. Residents must understand the purpose, development, and application of drug formularies and clinical guidelines. Discussion should include such issues as branding, generic drugs, off-label use, and use of free samples.

Systems-based Practice

Systems-based Practice includes behaviors that demonstrate an awareness of and responsiveness to the larger context of health care and the ability to engage system resources to provide care that is of optimal value. The following principles of Systems-based Practice apply to relationships with industry:

1. Sponsoring institutions and programs must develop policies to assure that clinical skills and judgment are learned in objective and evidence-based clinical and teaching environments free from inappropriate influence. These policies must clarify the differences between education and promotion.
2. Teaching institutions must ensure that programs have sufficient funds from appropriate sources to conduct their educational activities.
3. Resident curricula should include how to apply appropriate considerations of cost-benefit analysis as a component of prescribing practice.
4. Advocacy for patient rights within health care systems should include attention to pharmaceutical costs.

Interpersonal and Communication Skills

Interpersonal and Communication Skills provide the foundation upon which the satisfactory relationship between doctor and patient central to medicine is established. With regard to relationships with industry, particular aspects of Interpersonal and Communication Skills should be fostered through application of the following principles:

1. Resident curricula should include discussion and reflection on managing encounters with industry representatives.
2. Illustrative cases of how to handle patient requests for medication, particularly with regard to direct-to-consumer advertising of drugs, should be included in communication skills curricula.

Conclusion

The principles outlined in the previous paragraphs cannot guarantee individual or institutional professional behavior. Evidence exists, however, that policies relating to sources of educational support appear to affect what physicians believe and how they behave [24]. The value of these principles, therefore, lies in their ability to inform policy and to represent to the public the integrity and objectivity of the professional relationships expected by residency programs and their sponsoring institutions. The ultimate goal of these relationships is to foster effective Patient Care, the general competency that underlies the mission of medical education.

Inappropriate promotional activities by industry seriously compromise the professional relationships maintained by residents, faculty, and patients that form the substance of medicine. These inappropriate activities must not be allowed to continue where they exist. The interests of the patient must be paramount and not contaminated by the profit-driven interests of industry for their shareholders. Residency programs and their sponsoring institutions must teach and model core values that are demonstrated by the general competencies. The public and the profession look to teaching institutions to demonstrate particular clarity around issues of patient advocacy, complete and unbiased medical knowledge, and the application of that knowledge to continually improve the practice of medicine.

References

1. The Pharmaceutical Research and Manufacturers of America (PhRMA). New medicines new hope (annual report). 2001–2002. Available from URL: www.phrma/org.publications/publications/annual2001. Accessed 10/18/01.

2. Wazana A. Physicians and the pharmaceutical industry: is a gift ever just a gift? JAMA 2000 Jan 19; 283(3):373–80.

3. Hammond C. In the business. Endeavors. University of North Carolina at Chapel Hill: 1999. Available from URL: http://research.unc.edu/endeavors/fall99/business.htm. Accessed 01/03/02.

4. Ross J, Lurie P, Wolfe S. Medical education service suppliers: a threat to physician education. Public Citizen's Health Research Group 2000 July 19. Available from URL: http://www.citizen.org/publications/release.cfm?ID=7142. Accessed 01/14/02.

5. Rennie D. Thyroid storm. JAMA 1997 April 16; 277(15):1238–43.

6. Relman A. Separating continuing medical education from pharmaceutical marketing. JAMA 2001 Apr 18; 285(15):2009–12.

7. Chren M, Landefeld C. Physicians' behavior and their interactions with drug companies. JAMA 1994 Mar 2; 271(9):684–89.

8. Orlowski J, Wateska L. The effects of pharmaceutical firm enticements on physician prescribing patterns. there's no such thing as a free lunch. Chest 1992; 102:270–73.

9. Hafferty F. Beyond curriculum reform: confronting medicine's hidden curriculum. Acad Med 1998 April 73(4):403–7.

10. Stern D. In search of the informal curriculum: when and where professional values are taught. Acad Med 1998 Oct 73(10 Suppl 1):S-28–30.

11. Rothman D. Medical professionalism—focusing on the real issues. N Engl J Med 2000 342(17):1284–6.

12. Kassirer J. Financial indigestion. JAMA 2000 Nov 1; 284(17):2156–57.

13. Eichenwald K, Kolata G. Drug trials hide conflicts for doctors. NY Times 1999 May 16;Sect.1 (national).

14. Council on Ethical and Judicial Affairs. Gifts to physicians from industry. (E-8.061) American Medical Association (AMA). 2001. Available from URL: www.ama-assn.org/ama/pub/article/4001-4236.html. Accessed 10/30/01.

15. Coyle SL for the Ethics and Human Rights Committee, American College of Physicians—American Society of Internal Medicine. Physician-industry relations. Part 1: Individual physicians. Ann Intern Med 2002 March 5; 136(5):396–402.

16. Coyle SL for the Ethics and Human Rights Committee, American College of Physicians—American Society of Internal Medicine. Physician-industry relations. Part 2: Organizational issues. Ann Intern Med 2002 March 5; 136(5):403–6.

17. Canadian Medical Association (CMA). Physicians and the pharmaceutical industry. 2001. Available from URL: http://www.cma.ca/staticContent/HTML/N0/12/where we stand/physicians and the pharmaceutical industry.pdf. Accessed 01/03/02.

18. Accreditation Council for Continuing Medical Education (ACCME). Standards for Commercial Support of Continuing Medical Education. 2001 Available from URL: www.accme.org/pdfs/disclosure pol.pdf. Accessed 10/30/01.

19. Task Force on Financial Conflicts of Interest in Research. Protecting subjects, preserving trust, promoting progress: Policy and guidelines for the oversight of individual financial interests in human subjects research. Association of American Medical Colleges. 2002. Available from URL: http://www.aamc.org/members/coitf/firstreport.pdf. Accessed 3/11/02.

20. Accreditation Council for Graduate Medical Education (ACGME). General competencies. 2001. Available from URL: http://www.acgme. org/outcome/comp/compFull.asp. Accessed 10/16/01.

21. Kuczewski M. Developing competency in professionalism: the potential and the pitfalls. ACGME Bulletin 2001 October;3–6.

22. Arnold L. Assessing professionalism: from concept to construct. Acad Med. In press, 2001.

23. Ginsburg S, Regehr G, Hatala R, McNaughton N, Frohna A, Hodges B, et al. Context, conflict, and resolution: a new conceptual framework for evaluating professionalism. Acad Med 2000;75 Suppl: S6-11.

24. McCormick B, Tomlinson G, Brill-Edwards P, Detsky A. Effect of restricting contact between pharmaceutical company representatives and internal medicine residents on posttraining attitudes and behaviors. JAMA 2001 Oct 24/31; 286(16):1994–99.

Protecting Subjects, Preserving Trust,

Promoting Progress – Policy and Guidelines

for the Oversight of Individual Financial

Interests in Human Subjects Research

Task Force on Financial Conflicts of Interest in Clinical Research
December 2001

AAMC Task Force on Financial Conflicts of Interest In Clinical Research

Task Force Chair
William Danforth, M.D.
Chancellor Emeritus and
Vice-Chairman, Board of Trustees,
Washington University at
St. Louis

John Thomas Bigger, M.D.
Professor of Medicine and
Pharmacology, Columbia
University

Frank Davidoff, M.D.
Editor, *Annals of Internal
Medicine*

Martin J. Delaney
Founding Director, Project Inform

Susan Dentzer
NewsHour with Jim Lehrer

Susan H. Ehringhaus, Esq.
Vice Chancellor and General
Counsel, University of North
Carolina at Chapel Hill

Ginger Graham
Group Chairman, Guidant
Corporation

*Susan Hellmann, M.D., M.P.H.***
Chief Medical Officer, Genentech

Jeffrey Kahn, Ph.D., M.P.H.
Director, Center for Bioethics,
University of Minnesota

Marvin Kalb
Executive Director, Washington
Office, Joan Shorenstein Center for
the Press, Politics and Public
Policy, John F. Kennedy School of
Government

Russel E. Kaufman, M.D.
Vice Dean, Education and
Academic Affairs, Duke University
School of Medicine

Robert P. Kelch, M.D.
Dean, University of Iowa College
of Medicine

Mark R. Laret
Chief Executive Officer, University
of California, San Francisco
Medical Center

Joan S. Leonard, Esq.
Vice President and General
Counsel, Howard Hughes Medical
Institute

Ronald Levy, M.D.
Robert K. and Helen K. Summy
Professor in the School of
Medicine, Stanford University

Constance E. Lieber
President, NARSAD

Joseph B. Martin, M.D., Ph.D.
Dean, Faculty of Medicine,
Harvard Medical School

Edward D. Miller, M.D.
Dean, Johns Hopkins School of

Medicine; CEO, Johns Hopkins
Medicine

Thomas H. Murray, Ph.D.
President and Chief Executive
Officer, The Hastings Center

Charles P. O'Brien, M.D., Ph.D.
Chief of Psychiatry, Philadelphia
Veterans Affairs Medical Center;
Kenneth Appel Professor and
Vice-Chair of Psychiatry,
University of Pennsylvania

Hon. John E. Porter, Esq.
Partner
Hogan and Hartson, L.L.P.

Roger Porter, M.D.
Vice President Clinical Research
and Development, Wyeth-Ayerst
Research

Paul G. Ramsey, M.D.
Vice President for Medical Affairs
and Dean of the School of
Medicine, University of
Washington

Dorothy K. Robinson, Esq.
Vice President and General
Counsel, Yale University

Hedrick Smith∗
President Hedrick Smith
Productions, Inc.

Frances M. Visco, Esq.
President, The National Breast
Cancer Coalition

Savio Woo, Ph.D.
Director and Professor,
Institute for Gene Therapy,
Mount Sinai School of
Medicine

Alastair J.J. Wood, M.D.
Assistant Vice Chancellor for
Research, Professor of Medicine,
Professor of Pharmacology,
Vanderbilt University School of
Medicine

AAU LIAISON
Richard J. Turman
Director of Federal Relations,

The Association of American
Universities

AAMC STAFF
David Korn, M.D.
Senior Vice President,
Association of American
Medical Colleges Division of
Biomedical and Health Sciences
Research

Jennifer Kulynych, J.D., Ph.D.
Director, Association of American
Medical Colleges Division of
Biomedical and Health Sciences
Research

*Due to unanticipated professional obligations arising from the September 11th, 2001, attacks, Hedrick Smith was unable to participate in the drafting of this report.

**Susan Hellman, M.D., declines to endorse the report, primarily due to her concern that its recommendations present an impediment to research innovation.

The work of the Task Force was supported in part by a grant from the Howard Hughes Medical Institute.

Preface

In October of 2000, in a speech entitled *Trust Us to Make a Difference*, Dr. Jordan Cohen, President of the Association of American Medical Colleges (AAMC), announced the formation of a new Task Force on Conflicts of Interest in Clinical Research chaired by Dr. William Danforth, Chancellor Emeritus of Washington University of St. Louis.[1] Dr. Cohen charged this Task Force to respond to deepening

---

[1]   Cohen JJ. Trust us to make a difference: Ensuring public confidence in the integrity of clinical research. Acad. Med. 2001; 76:209–214.

public concern over researchers' perceived conflicts of interest by forging consensus principles and guidelines for the oversight of financial interests in research involving human subjects.

To achieve a broad consensus in support of new policy recommendations, the AAMC selected Task Force members not only from the leadership of academic medicine, but also from the ranks of prominent clinical investigators, patient representatives, former legislators, drug and device company executives, and journalists. The Task Force met in May and September of 2001 and engaged in consultation and extensive deliberations.[2] The first product of these efforts is this document, entitled *Guidelines for Developing and Implementing A Policy Concerning Individual Financial Interests in Research*. The 2001 *Guidelines* are intended to augment and impart greater specificity to the AAMC's 1990 *Guidelines for Dealing with Faculty Conflicts of Commitment and Conflicts of Interest in Research*.

In creating new guidance, Task Force members drew upon their varied experience as discoverers, developers, producers, and consumers of medical products, but remained focused on a shared objective: to preserve public trust in clinical research while sustaining medical progress. As a result, the 2001 *Guidelines* recommend policies that will strengthen the protection of human subjects, while enabling the robust, productive collaborations between industry and academic medicine that have developed in the past three decades and have contributed greatly to improvements in patient care and to the success of American medicine.

The 2001 *Guidelines* provide a model for baseline standards and practices in the oversight of financial interests in research. This guidance addresses the financial interests of individual faculty, staff,

---

[2] The Task Force acknowledges the prior efforts of a group of leaders from academic medicine who met in November of 2000 for a consensus conference moderated by Dr. Joseph B. Martin, Dean of the Faculty of Medicine at Harvard Medical School. The Consensus Statement produced by this group contains a number of the recommendations endorsed in the AAMC's 2001 *Guidelines*.

employees, students, fellows and trainees of our member institutions. Currently, the Task Force is considering principles for oversight of the financial interests that institutions and their officers may hold in human subjects research. Informed by these deliberations, the AAMC intends to issue a second guidance document on institutional financial interests in human subjects research within the coming year.

I. Introduction

Institutions in which faculty, staff, or students conduct research involving human subjects must ensure that the safety and welfare of those subjects and the integrity of the research are never subordinated to, or compromised by, financial interests or the pursuit of personal gain. The AAMC Task Force on Financial Conflicts of Interest in Clinical Research acknowledges significant ongoing public concern about the existence of financial interests in human subjects research, and strongly encourages academic institutions to respond in ways that instill confidence in their capacity to identify these interests and to manage them safely and effectively.

Competing interests, particularly those engendered by a desire to advance scientific knowledge or to achieve professional recognition, are an inescapable fact of academic life. Most are managed through institutional policies and practices, and through the constraints imposed by the scientific method.[3] Yet financial interests in human subjects research are distinct from other interests inherent in academic life that might impart bias or induce improper behavior, because financial interests are discretionary, and because the perception is widespread that they may entail special risks. Specifically, opportunities to profit from research may affect – or appear to affect – a researcher's judgements about which subjects to enroll, the clinical care provided to subjects, even the proper use of subjects' confidential health information. Financial interests also threaten scientific integrity when they foster real or apparent biases in study design,

---

[3] D. Korn, Conflicts of interest in biomedical research. JAMA 2000; 284: 2234–2237.

data collection and analysis, adverse event reporting, or the presentation and publication of research findings.

At the same time, a principled partnership between industry and academia is essential if we are to preserve medical progress and to continue to improve the health of our citizenry. The generous public support of scientific research in America's universities since World War II has been predicated on the expectation that scientific advancements will yield tangible public benefits – a robust economy, strong national security, and a healthy citizenry. Yet, public research support is, for the most part, purposefully limited in scope to basic research, and essentially ceases at the point at which scientific invention enters the pathway of product development. In biomedicine, with rare exceptions, it is the private sector, not academia, that develops diagnostic, therapeutic, and preventative products and brings them to market. At the crucial interface between innovation and development, researchers from academic medicine often play a critical role by conducting the early translational research that gives rise to new products, and by testing these novel products for safety and efficacy.

As the AAMC first noted in its 1990 *Guidelines for Dealing with Faculty Conflicts of Commitment and Conflicts of Interest in Research*, the opportunity for researchers to receive financial rewards from these endeavors is not intrinsically unacceptable, as long as this opportunity does not adversely influence scientific or clinical decision-making. Importantly, however, though a researcher may strive to insulate his or her decision-making from bias, the mere appearance of a conflict between financial interests and professional responsibilities may weaken public confidence in the researcher's objectivity. The real and apparent risks posed by financial interests likewise have the potential to threaten public support for the research mission of academic institutions. The credibility of academic medicine – and the public trust we prize so highly – could be undermined by revelations that an institution has failed to exercise rigorous oversight of financial interests in human subjects research and may thereby have exposed research subjects to avoidable harms.

Because the safety and welfare of human beings are at stake, financial interests in human subjects research are rightly the focus of intense scrutiny. Renewed attention to what are often termed "financial conflicts of interest" is occurring at a time when academic medical institutions are turning increasingly to private funds as a source of support for clinical research. Moreover, current federal policies encourage institutions to seek private investment as a vehicle for translating academic biomedical research into medically useful products. Under the regulations implementing the Bayh-Dole Act of 1980,[4] institutions and researchers are to share in the return on successful inventions arising from federally-funded research.

Bayh-Dole is widely viewed as having created incentives for socially useful collaboration between academia and industry. The resulting commercialization of research harnesses the collective intellectual and creative talents of university faculty, speeds the development of new and improved therapies, stimulates regional economic growth, and contributes to the economic viability of research institutions.[5] Notwithstanding these benefits, the increasing involvement of academics in commercially-sponsored research places new demands on institutions to be scrupulous in crafting and enforcing their conflict of interest policies, and on investigators to be diligent in adhering to them.

Current federal regulations concerning financial interests in research were intended to promote objectivity in federally-funded research and to ensure the reliability of data submitted to the Food and Drug Administration (FDA) – not to protect human subjects *per se*.[6]

---

4   "Rights to Inventions Made by Nonprofit Organizations and Small Business Firms," codified at 37 CFR Part 401.

5   University-Industry Research Collaboration Initiative of the Business-Higher Education Forum, *Working Together, Creating Knowledge: The University-Industry Research Collaboration Initiative* (June 2001).

6   The PHS regulations are found at 42 C.F.R. Subpart F, the FDA regulations at 21 C.F.R. Parts 54, 312, 314, 320, 330, 601, 807, 812, 814, and

Under these regulations, institutions applying for Public Health Service (PHS) funding[7] must solicit annual financial disclosure statements from each investigator who plans to participate in PHS-funded research, review these statements for evidence of a "significant financial interest" that "would reasonably appear to be affected by the research," and then "manage, reduce, or eliminate" the interest within 60 days.[8] Institutions must report to the funding agency the existence, though not the nature or details, of any "conflicting" financial interest that the institution determines could directly and significantly affect the research, and assure the funding agency that the interest has been appropriately managed, reduced, or eliminated.[9]

In 1999 the FDA adopted financial disclosure regulations that require parties who submit applications for approval of a new drug, device, or biological product to provide certain information about financial relationships between sponsors and investigators. Typically academic institutions are not required to collect this information;

---

860. The National Science Foundation has adopted a financial disclosure policy that is similar to that of the PHS. 60 Fed. Reg. 132, 35809 (July 11, 1995).

[7] This includes all institutions seeking research grants from the National Institutes of Health, a PHS agency.

[8] The PHS regulations define a "significant financial interest" as "anything of monetary value" except for the following: salary, royalties, or other remuneration from the institution; ownership interests in institutional applicants for SBIR grants; income from public or non-profit sources for lecturing, teaching, or serving on advisory boards or review panels; equity interests that do not exceed $10,000 or 5% ownership of a single entity; or other payments that in the aggregate are not expected to exceed $10,000 during the next 12 months. 42 C.F.R. §50.603.

[9] The regulations state that a conflict of interest exists "when the designated official(s) reasonably determines that a Significant Financial Interest could directly and significantly affect the design, conduct, or reporting of the PHS-funded research." 42 C.F.R. § 50.605.

instead, the responsibility rests with the sponsoring company.[10] FDA's regulations for marketing applicants differ from the rules that apply to recipients of PHS research funds in important to the agency once the research is complete and the data are submitted in a marketing application; FDA exempts a greater dollar amount from the disclosure obligation; and FDA's disclosure obligation is narrower, applying only to certain "covered clinical studies" and requiring the applicant to submit only information about the investigator's financial interests in the research sponsor.

What the existing federal financial disclosure regulations *do not* require is a comprehensive system of disclosure and oversight, pursuant to which institutions would collect and carefully review information on all significant financial interests in human subjects research, whether such research is federally-funded or respects: the FDA requirements are retrospective, meaning that financial interests must only be reported privately sponsored. Equally important, federal financial disclosure regulations do not mandate special scrutiny of financial interests in human subjects research, nor do they acknowledge the unique obligations that attend research involving human beings.

Mindful of these obligations, the Task Force asserts that academic medicine must look beyond the scope of current federal financial disclosure requirements and delineate more fully the bounds of acceptable conduct for those who conduct research with human subjects. Some institutions have made exemplary efforts in this regard. For others, revising policies and practices in the manner that we recommend

---

[10] The exception would occur when an academic institution holds the investigational new drug (IND) application or investigational device exemption (IDE) for the product studied in the research. FDA has stated that in this circumstance, the IND or IDE holder must collect financial disclosure information for the benefit of the party who will eventually file the marketing application. Food and Drug Administration, Guidance: Financial Disclosure by Clinical Investigators (March 20, 2001) <available at http://www.fda.gov/oc/guidance/financialdis. html>.

might require a significant investment of time and resources, and perhaps a discomfiting change in institutional culture. We are convinced nonetheless that all institutions can rise to this challenge. These 2001 *Guidelines for Developing and Implementing a Policy Concerning Individual Financial Interests in Human Subjects Research* are evidence of our collective willingness to seek, to merit, and to sustain public trust in the research mission of academic medicine.

Core Principles to Guide Policy Development

This document offers guidance to institutions in their efforts to provide responsible and effective oversight of financial interests in human subjects research. Academic institutions share common concerns, yet each retains its own unique culture and mode of self-governance. Institutional procedures for the oversight of financial interests in research will vary accordingly. These guidelines create a model for baseline standards and practices, without limiting the prerogative of institutions to implement conflict of interest policies in a manner best suited to local needs. The Task Force recognizes that some institutions may determine that additional restrictions are appropriate. Likewise, we do not discourage institutional variations in process or in the allocation of the oversight responsibilities described in this guidance, provided that the review and management functions that we advocate are performed fully.

As a starting point, we emphasize that the Task Force does not assume that financial interests in human subjects research are categorically improper, or that those who hold such interests cannot conduct research with the requisite scientific objectivity and integrity or protect the welfare of human research subjects. Recognizing, however, that research with human subjects is a privilege that imposes unique obligations, the Task Force believes that the following principles should animate institutional policies concerning financial interests in such research:

   A. With the welfare of research subjects always of foremost concern,
      an institution should regard all significant financial interests in

human subjects research as potentially problematic and, therefore, as requiring close scrutiny. Institutional policies should establish the rebuttable presumption that an individual who holds a significant financial interest in research involving human subjects may not conduct such research. The intent is not to suggest that every financial interest jeopardizes the welfare of human subjects or the integrity of research, but rather to ensure that institutions systematically review any financial interest that might give rise to the perception of a conflict of interest, and further, that they limit the conduct of human subjects research by financially interested individuals to those situations in which the circumstances are compelling. The presumption against significant financial interests in human subjects research should apply whether the research is funded by a public agency, a non-profit entity, or a commercial sponsor, and wherever the research may be carried out.

B. In the event of compelling circumstances, an individual holding significant financial interests in human subjects research may be permitted to conduct the research. Whether the circumstances are deemed compelling will depend in each case upon the nature of the science, the nature of the interest, how closely the interest is related to the research, and the degree to which the interest may be affected by the research. When the financial interest is directly related to the research and may be substantially affected by it (e.g., an equity interest in a start-up company that manufactures the investigational product), the risk is greatest and the bar must be high; however, even direct and potentially lucrative financial interests may be justified in some circumstances. For example, when the individual holding such interests is uniquely qualified by virtue of expertise and experience and the research could not otherwise be conducted as safely or effectively without that individual, he or she should be permitted the opportunity to rebut the presumption against financial interests by demonstrating these facts to the satisfaction of an institution's conflict of interest (COI) committee.[11] The COI committee might approve the involvement of such an individual in the research, subject to conditions that ensure effective management of the conflict and credible oversight of the research.[12]

C. Institutional policies should require full *prior reporting* of each covered individual's significant financial interests that would reasonably appear to be affected by the individual's research, *updated reporting* of any relevant change in financial circumstances, and *review* of any significant financial interests in a research project by the institution's COI committee *prior to final IRB approval of*

---

[11] The Task Force recognizes that institutional practices may differ in their allocation of responsibilities for COI reviews between designated committees and officials, and that in some institutions an IRB may perform a substantive review of financial conflicts of interest. The Task Force strongly recommends that the COI process be separate from the IRB, although with clear channels of communication between them. In all cases the same rebuttable presumption against the financial interest should apply, and the financially interested individual should be given the opportunity to demonstrate "compelling circumstances" to the cognizant authority.

[12] To illustrate, the inventor of an implantable medical device, who under the Bayh-Dole Act might receive royalty income, and who might also be compensated by the device manufacturer for training other physicians to use the device, may also be the individual who is best qualified to implant the device in human subjects safely under experimental conditions. The COI committee might, at its discretion, agree to permit this financially-interested inventor to participate in a clinical study of the device at the institution, subject to management conditions crafted to minimize the potential conflict of interest. These conditions could include, in addition to full disclosure of the interest (to research subjects and others as described in this guidance), requirements that informed consent be obtained by a clinician with no financial ties to the research, and that the research be overseen by a monitoring board.

the research. COI committee findings and determinations should inform the IRB's review of any research protocol or proposal, although the IRB may require additional safeguards or demand reduction or elimination of the financial interest. The Task Force recommends that, as between the COI committee and the IRB, the more stringent determination should be dispositive. Institutional policies should *specify which responsible institutional officials are empowered to make final and binding decisions* about who may conduct IRB-approved research.

D. Institutional policies governing financial interests in human subjects research should be comprehensive, unambiguous, well-publicized, consistently applied, and enforced through effective sanctions. Moreover, in today's research environment, which is both increasingly entrepreneurial and subject to intense public scrutiny, *transparency* must be the watchword for the oversight of financial interests. Transparency is achieved through full and ongoing internal reporting and external disclosure of significant financial interests that would reasonably appear to affect the welfare of subjects or the conduct or communication of research.

E. Transparency, though necessary to sustain public confidence in academic research, is not sufficient to protect human subjects. When an institution finds that financial interests in human subjects research are justified by compelling circumstances, those interests and the research in question must be managed through *rigorous, effective, and disinterested monitoring* undertaken by individuals with no financial or professional ties to the research or direct reporting relationships to the researchers. Approaches to monitoring might include the following: regular audits of the informed consent and enrollment process, the involvement of a patient representative or ombudsman when subjects are recruited and informed consent is obtained, a requirement to escrow the financial interest until the investigational product has been approved and on the market for a specified time period, and the use of data safety monitoring boards. In some circumstances monitoring boards might be composed wholly of institutional representatives; however, when the institution itself holds a financial interest in the research, disinterested monitoring might require the participation of individuals from outside the institution.

F. Institutions and individual faculty, staff, employees, students, fellows, and trainees *bear a shared responsibility* for the oversight of financial interests in human subjects research, *yet each remains accountable* for the effectiveness of the oversight system. Individuals who conduct human subjects research must familiarize themselves with their institutions' COI policies and act diligently to fulfil the requirements imposed by these policies.

II. Policy Guidelines

An institutional policy on individual financial interests in human subjects research should be consistent with PHS regulations, and should contain the following elements:

Definitions of key terms.

A description of the *scope and substantive requirements* of the policy.

A description of *the process by which covered individuals will report significant financial interests in human subjects research* to institutional officials.

A description of the *process by which financial reports will be reviewed* by institutional officials (e.g., the institution's COI committee).

A description of the *criteria the COI committee will apply* to determine *whether a "financially interested individual" has demonstrated compelling circumstances that justify allowing that individual to conduct human subjects research.*

A description of the *process by which summary information concerning the nature and amount of any significant financial interest* in human subjects research, *COI committee determinations* concerning that interest, and *any conditions or management plan* will be *reported* to IRBs and to appropriate institutional officials.

A description of the *process by which significant financial interests* in human subjects research *will be disclosed* to research subjects,

editors of publications, the public, and as otherwise required by
the policy.

A description of the *process by which* the institution will *implement*
and *monitor compliance* with the policy.

A description of the *sanctions* to be imposed for violations of the
policy and the *procedures for adjudication and appeal*.

A. Definitions

Compelling Circumstances are those facts that convince the
institution's COI committee that a financially interested individual should be permitted to conduct human subjects research.
When considering a request by a financially-interested individual to conduct human subjects research, the circumstances that
the COI committee should evaluate include the nature of the
research, the magnitude of the interest and the degree to which
it is related to the research, the extent to which the interest could
be directly and substantially affected by the research, and the
degree of risk to the human subjects involved that is inherent in
the research protocol. The committee should also consider the
extent to which the interest is amenable to effective oversight
and management.

Conducting Research means, with respect to a research protocol,
designing research, directing research or serving as the principal
investigator, enrolling research subjects (including obtaining subjects' informed consent) or making decisions related to eligibility
to participate in research, analyzing or reporting research data, or
submitting manuscripts concerning the research for publication.

Covered Individual includes any faculty (fully-, partially-, or non-
salaried) or faculty agent, staff, student, fellow, trainee, or administrator who, under the aegis of the institution or pursuant to the review
and approval of the institution's IRB, conducts research involving
human subjects.

Disclosure means a release of relevant information about significant financial interests in human subjects research to parties outside

the institution's COI review and management processes (e.g., to research subjects or journal editors).

Financially Interested Company means a commercial entity with financial interests that would reasonably appear to be affected by the conduct or outcome of the research.[13] This term includes companies that compete with the sponsor of the research or the manufacturer of the investigational product, if the covered individual actually knows that the financial interests of such a company would reasonably appear to be affected by the research. This term also includes any entity acting as the agent of a financially interested company (e.g., a contract research organization).

Financially Interested Individual means a covered individual who holds a significant financial interest that would reasonably appear to be affected by the individual's human subjects research. Human Subjects Research includes *all* research meeting the definition of "research" performed with "human subjects" as these terms are defined in the federal Common Rule (45 C.F.R. Part 46 and 21 C.F.R. Part 56), regardless of the source of research funding or whether the research is otherwise subject to federal regulation. In the event that the Common Rule definitions of "human subjects" or "research" are modified through rulemaking, any such revisions shall apply for the purposes of this guidance.

Rebuttable Presumption Against Financial Interests in Human Subjects Research means the institution will presume, in order to assure that all potentially problematic circumstances are reviewed, that a financially interested individual may not conduct the human subjects research in question. This rule is not intended to be

---

[13] Under the standard articulated in the PHS regulations, institutions must solicit and review information about investigators' significant financial interests in any entity "whose financial interests would reasonably appear to be affected by the [PHS-funded] research." 42 C.F.R. §50.604(c)(1)(ii).

absolute: a financially interested individual may rebut the presumption by demonstrating facts that, in the opinion of the COI committee, constitute compelling circumstances. The individual would then be allowed to conduct the research under conditions specified by the COI committee and approved by the responsible IRB.

Reporting means the provision of information about significant financial interests in human subjects research by a covered individual to responsible institutional officials and to the institutional COI committee, or the transmission of such information within institutional channels (e.g., from the COI committee to the IRB).

Responsible Institutional Official means a Dean, Provost, CEO, or other institutional official who is responsible for the oversight of research programs within the institution.

Responsible IRB is the institutional review board (or boards) with jurisdiction over the research as specified in the multiple projects assurance (MPA) (or the federal-wide assurance (FWA)) that the institution has provided to the U.S. Department of Health and Human Services, or as otherwise established under DHHS or FDA regulation or policy.

Significant Financial Interests in Research include the following interests of the covered individual (and his or her spouse and dependent children), or of any foundation or entity controlled or directed by the individual or his or her spouse:

> Consulting fees, honoraria (including honoraria from a third party, if the original source is a financially interested company), gifts or other emoluments, or "in kind" compensation from a financially interested company (or entitlement to the same), whether for consulting, lecturing, travel, service on an advisory board, or for any other purpose not directly related to the reasonable costs of conducting the research (as specified in the research agreement), that in the aggregate have in the prior calendar year exceeded the de minimis amount established in PHS regulation (presently $10,000), or are expected to exceed that amount in the next twelve months.

Equity interests, including stock options, of any amount in a non-publicly-traded financially interested company (or entitlement to the same).

Equity interests (or entitlement to the same) in a publicly-traded financially interested company that exceed the defined de minimis amount (see exceptions below).

Royalty income or the right to receive future royalties under a patent license or copyright, where the research is directly related to the licensed technology or work.[14]

Any non-royalty payments or entitlements to payments in connection with the research that are not directly related to the reasonable costs of the research (as specified in the research agreement between the sponsor and the institution). This includes any bonus or milestone payments to the investigators in excess of reasonable costs incurred, whether such payments are received from a financially interested company or from the institution (note *prohibition* in B(11) on milestone payments tied to the achievement of particular research results).

Service as an officer, director, or in any other fiduciary role for a financially interested company, whether or not remuneration is received for such service.

Exceptions. Significant financial interests in research *do not include* the following:

Interests of any amount in publicly traded, diversified mutual funds.

Stock in a publicly-traded company that (when valued in reference to current public prices) meets the de minimis criteria

---

[14] When evaluating future royalty interests, in addition to the factors listed in the definition of compelling circum-stances, the COI committee might consider the anticipated time interval between the research and marketing approval of the investigational product.

established in PHS financial disclosure regulations (presently, an interest that does not exceed $10,000 in value and does not represent more than a 5% ownership interest in any single entity).

Stock options in a publicly-traded company that (when valued using accepted valuation methods) meet the de minimis criteria established in PHS financial disclosure regulations (presently, an interest that does not exceed $10,000 in value and does not represent more than a 5% ownership interest in any single entity).

Payments to the institution, or via the institution to the individual, that are directly related to reasonable costs incurred in the conduct of research as specified in the research agreement(s) between the sponsor and the institution.

Salary and other payments for services from the institution.

B. Scope and Substance of Policy

1. Conflict of Interest (COI) Official and Committee. Federal regulations require PHS-funded institutions to appoint a COI official to review financial interests in PHS-sponsored research.[15] The Task Force recommends that institutions also establish a standing COI committee.[16] COI committee membership should include individuals who conduct human subjects research at the institution, as well as the institution's COI official and other officials experienced in the oversight of conflicts of interest and familiar with applicable laws and regulations. A liaison to the IRB is recommended. Institutions might also consider means of involving community or patient representatives in the COI oversight process.

---

[15]   42 C.F.R. § 50.604(b).

[16]   References in this guidance to the "institution's COI committee" apply to the institution's COI official in the event that an institution chooses not to establish a standing COI committee.

Institutions should ensure that the COI committee responsibilities include the following:

a. *Review* of any request by a financially interested individual to rebut the presumption that he or she may not conduct human subjects research.

b. *Documentation* of the committee's findings and the bases for any recommendation to permit or to recommend against permitting a financially interested individual to conduct human subjects research. In either case the COI committee should prepare a summary report describing the nature and amount of the financial interest and the committee's recommendations. This summary report should be made available to the IRB. When the COI committee has recommended that a financially interested individual be permitted to conduct human subjects research and the IRB has approved the research and the individual's participation, the summary report should be provided to research subjects or the public, upon request.

c. *Management and oversight* when a financially interested individual is permitted to conduct human subjects research. As a first principle, the COI committee should encourage the financially interested individual to minimize the potential for conflict of interest by reducing or eliminating the interest or the individual's direct involvement in the research. The COI committee should specify the monitoring procedures or other conditions to be imposed when a financially interested individual will be permitted to conduct human subjects research.

d. *Communication* to the IRB, and to responsible institutional officials, of summary information about the nature and amount of any significant financial interest in human subjects research, along with the committee's findings and recommendations concerning requests by financially interested individuals to conduct such research.

2. Process. Every institution should adopt mechanisms that ensure the following:

a. The financial reports of covered individuals are collected and maintained in a format that is readily accessible to the COI committee and responsible institutional officials;

b. The responsible IRB and responsible institutional officials are alerted whenever a financially interested individual proposes to conduct human subjects research;

c. Prior to the IRB's final approval (whether initial or continuing approval) of human subjects research, the COI committee has informed the IRB and responsible institutional officials of any significant financial interests held by financially interested individuals who will conduct the research, as well as the COI committee's findings and recommendations concerning the same;

d. Financially interested individuals are provided an avenue for appealing decisions of the COI committee; and

e. When financially interested individuals will be permitted to conduct human subjects research, the financial interests in question are disclosed in accordance with the institution's COI policies.

1. Written Policy. Every institution engaged in human subjects research should have a written policy on financial interests in such research. This policy should define all key terms clearly and should detail substantive prohibitions and restrictions, as well as the procedures for reporting financial interests, reviewing financial reports, disclosing reported information, implementing the policy, appealing decisions concerning the policy, and sanctioning non-compliance with the policy. The written policy should explain the criteria that the COI committee will apply when reviewing a request by a financially interested individual to rebut the presumption that he or she may not conduct human subjects research. The policy and related

information should be readily accessible to covered individuals and to the public; in addition to conventional means of communication, the policy should be placed on the institution's website, if one exists.

☐ 4. Rebuttable Presumption that Financially Interested Individuals May Not Conduct Human Subjects Research. The policy should establish the presumption that, in the absence of compelling circumstances, a financially interested individual may not conduct human subjects research. This presumption should be rebuttable when compelling circumstances exist.

☐ a. The policy should allow the COI committee, after it reviews the relevant facts and circumstances and documents the compelling circumstances, to recommend that a financially interested individual be permitted to conduct the research, and to make recommendations for appropriate monitoring and oversight.

☐ b. A summary report indicating the nature and amount of the financial interest and COI committee recommendations should be transmitted to the responsible IRB and to responsible institutional officials.

1. Monitoring. The policy should specify procedures for internal, and, when deemed necessary, external monitoring when a financially interested individual is permitted to conduct human subjects research.

☐ 6. Reporting by Covered Individuals. The policy should require covered individuals to report to the institution all significant financial interests that would reasonably appear to be affected by the individual's current or anticipated human subjects research. In making such reports, each covered individual should be required to declare explicitly whether he or she does or does not have such financial interests; the failure to report is unacceptable.

☐ a. Reports should be required at least annually, with prompt updating whenever there is an interim, material change in significant financial interests.

☐ b. Some institutions currently require a researcher to indicate on the institutional face sheet accompanying the research proposal whether the researcher holds any significant financial interest in the research. All institutions should consider adopting this practice for research involving human subjects.

2. Reporting to Supervisor. When the COI committee determines that a financially-interested individual should be permitted to conduct human subjects research, a copy of the committee's summary report describing the financial interest and any conditions to be imposed upon the research should be provided to the head of the unit (e.g., department chair) in which the covered individual resides adminis- tratively, and to the responsible dean, provost, CEO, or other official who has institutional responsibility for monitoring the activities of the covered individual.

3. Investigator Certification to IRB. When a research proposal is sub- mitted to the IRB for review, including continuing review (where applicable), each covered individual who will conduct the research should attest in writing to the IRB that financial report information on file for that individual is current and will be updated promptly to reflect relevant changes in financial circumstances. The IRB should forward any information that it receives concerning a sig- nificant financial interest in human subjects research to the COI committee.

4. COI Committee Review of Significant Financial Interest Created by Licensing Agreements. Prior to executing a technology licens- ing agreement, the Office of Technology Licensing must determine whether the agreement would create a significant individual finan- cial interest in ongoing or proposed human subjects research, and if so, inform the institution's COI committee of the proposed terms of the agreement. The COI committee should either approve the conduct of the research by the individual who will hold the financial interest, subject to an appropriate monitoring plan, or determine that the individual may not conduct the research if he or she wishes to retain the financial interest.

10. Disclosure of Significant Financial Interests.

☐ a. The policy should require disclosure of the existence of significant financial interests in human subjects research as follows: to state and federal officials, as required by statute or regulation; to research funders or sponsors; to the editors of any publication to which a covered individual submits a manuscript concerning the research;[17] and in any substantive public communication of the research results, whether oral or written.

☐ b. If an institution participating in a multi-center trial has judged a financially-interested individual eligible to conduct human subjects research at its site, that fact should be made known to the Principal Investigator or Sponsor, and to the IRBs of other institutions participating in the trial.

☐ c. Research consent forms should, as a matter of institution's COI policy, disclose the existence of any significant financial interest held by a covered individual who is conducting the human subjects research. The precise wording of disclosure in the consent form should be determined by the IRB, but should include an explanation of the fact that the financial interest in question has been reviewed by the COI committee, approved subject to committee over-sight, and determined by both the committee and the IRB not to pose any additional significant risk to the welfare of research subjects or the integrity of the research.

☐ d. If the institution's COI committee has authorized a financially interested individual to conduct human subjects research, the disclosure statement in the research consent form should indicate

---

[17] Disclosure to journal editors should take the form of an affirmative statement on behalf of each covered individual who conducted the research that he or she either does or does not hold significant financial interests in the research. This requirement is consistent with the recent uniform disclosure requirements published by a group of editors of major medical journals. F. Davidoff, C. D. DeAngelis, J.M. Drazen, et al. Sponsorship, authorship, and accountability. JAMA; 286;10:1232–1234.

that additional information (to include the COI summary report describing the nature and amouont of the financial interest) will be provided to research subjects upon request.[18]

11. Prohibition on Payments for Results. The policy should prohibit payments from the institution or the sponsor to a covered individual, if such payments are conditioned upon a particular research result or are tied to successful research outcomes. Payments for subject enrollment or for referral of patients to research studies should be permitted only to the extent that such payments:

☐ a. Are reasonably related to costs incurred, as specified in the research agreement between the sponsor and the institution;

☐ b. Reflect the fair market value of services performed; and

☐ c. Are commensurate with the efforts of the individual(s) performing the research.

12. Affirmation of Institutional Policies on Intellectual Property and Publication Rights. The COI policy should affirm an investigator's accountability for the integrity of any publication that bears his or her name. The policy should also affirm the right of a principal investigator to receive, analyze, and interpret all data generated in the research, and to publish the results, independent of the outcome of the research. Institutions should not enter, nor permit a covered individual to enter, research agreements that permit a sponsor or other financially interested company to require more than a reasonable period of pre-publication review,[19] or that interfere with

---

[18]   The National Human Research Protections Advisory Commission has recommended this approach to the disclosure of researchers' financial interests to research subjects. Letter from Mary Faith Marshall, Ph.D., Chair, NHRPAC, to Assistant Surgeon General/Acting Principal Deputy Assistant Secretary for Health Arthur J. Lawrence, Ph.D., dated August 23, 2001.

[19]   For sponsored research, a reasonable period of review would be no more than 90 days, unless both parties agree that extenuating circumstances

an investigator's access to the data or ability to analyze the data independently.[20]

1. Protection of Students and Trainees. Commercially sponsored research may give rise to financial incentives that conflict with a supervising researcher's responsibility to foster the academic development of students and trainees. Agreements with sponsors or financially interested companies that place restrictions on the activities of students or trainees or that bind students or trainees to non-disclosure provisions should ordinarily be prohibited. When deemed unavoidable, such agreements should be subjected to close scrutiny by the responsible university official and the institution's COI committee, and should be fully disclosed to all students and trainees prior to their involvement in the research. Under no circumstance should a student or trainee be permitted to participate in research if the terms and conditions of participation would prevent him or her from meeting applicable institutional degree requirements (e.g., completion and public defense of a thesis or dissertation). The institution's policy on financial interests in research should reaffirm, or explicitly cross-reference, the relevant institutional documents that address these matters.

2. Legal Obligations. The policy documents should alert covered individuals to all state and federal requirements applicable to financial interests in research, including state financial disclosure laws (if applicable), state licensure and professional conduct standards relevant to

---

require an extension of time. The Task Force notes that for research involving NIH-funded research tools, the NIH has stated that it would consider a 30–60 day review period to be reasonable. National Institutes of Health, Principles and Guidelines for Recipients of NIH Research Grants and Contract on Obtaining and Disseminating

[20] When research involves more than one institution and numerous investigators (e.g., a multi-center trial), the investigators may delegate primary authorship to a subset who will take responsibility for the publication.

conflict of interest, federal laws relative to "finders fees" for research subjects, and SEC prohibitions against insider trading. The policy should also direct investigators who conduct FDA-regulated research to familiarize themselves with FDA policies concerning promotional activities.

3. Sanctions. The policy should define the range of possible sanctions for non-compliance, up to and including dismissal. The policy should reference the procedures to be followed for sanctioning violations and for appealing adverse determinations.

C. Policy Implementation

1. Information Flow. Institutions should implement policies, procedures, and systems that will facilitate prompt reporting of significant financial interests to the institution and enable the timely flow of accurate and complete information to and from the COI committee, the responsible IRB(s), the institutional Office of Technology Licensing, and responsible institutional officials.

   1. Electronic Reporting Form. To enhance the efficiency of the reporting process, institutions should consider adopting an electronic disclosure form and permitting covered individuals to make and update financial reports on-line and in real time.

   2. Resources. Implementation of a comprehensive, effective COI policy may require institutions to devote new resources to their compliance effort. Institutions should ensure that adequate resources and personnel are allocated to support effective, credible oversight of financial interests in human subjects research.

   3. Written Acknowledgement Required. Institutions should require that all individuals who conduct human subjects research read and acknowledge in writing that they understand and agree to comply with the institution's COI policies.

   4. Education and Training. Institutions should adopt mechanisms for disseminating COI policies to all faculty, staff, students, and trainees, and for providing appropriate education and training in these policies.

5. Compliance Monitoring. Institutions should regularly assess compliance with COI policies through the use of internal audit mechanisms and other appropriate self-evaluation strategies.
6. Accreditation. The effectiveness of COI policies and a formal assessment of institution-wide compliance with these policies should be examined as an element of any accreditation process for the institution's human subjects protection program.

Epilogue

During the past two decades, remarkable advancements in biomedical research and the stimulus of the Bayh-Dole Act have vastly increased the breadth and depth of engagement of academic medicine with industry. The growth of the biotechnology industry is a celebrated accomplishment of the U.S. economy during the second half of the 20th century, and together with the information technology industry has spurred public perception of research universities as engines of economic development and social betterment. But at the same time, the public insists that universities remain unblemished by financial self-interest and continue to serve society as trusted and impartial arbiters of knowledge. This "conflict of public expectations" is nowhere more intense than in academic medicine and in research involving human subjects, where the steadily deepening engagement of clinical research with the world of commerce is seen by many influential observers as threatening both research integrity and the welfare of research participants.

The Task Force acknowledges the enormous benefits that have inured to the public from the commercial development of medical inventions made in academic medical centers and anticipates that the relationships of these centers with industry will only continue to deepen in an era in which terms like genomics, proteomics, and physiomics are becoming commonplace. But the Task Force also recognizes that the public's extraordinary support of academic biomedical research will remain critically dependent upon public confidence and trust that are especially vulnerable in research involving human subjects. This is the reality, and it must be appreciated by industry as much as by academe if their future interactions are to thrive.

This first report from the AAMC Task Force on Financial Conflicts of Interest in Clinical Research deals with individual financial interests. It intends to raise the standards of institutional oversight and management of financial conflicts of interest, and make them more uniform across academic medicine. The report respects institutional autonomy: the recommended policy and guidance provide a floor that permits institutions to adopt even more stringent provisions if they wish. The report eschews a "one size fits all approach:" it recognizes that each case of potential financial conflict of interest in research must be closely examined on its merits, and must respect the particular institutional, individual, and scientific circumstances that may attend it.

The Task Force does not believe, and does not intend, that adoption of the recommended policy and guidelines by the academic medical community should interfere with healthy academic–industry relationships or with the continued robust flow of academic biomedical invention into beneficial products. The Task Force does believe that these policies and guidance can help to ensure that the relationships remain principled, protective of research subjects and scientific integrity, and capable of withstanding intense public scrutiny.

Protecting Subjects, Preserving Trust, Promoting Progress II: Principles and Recommendations for Oversight of an Institution's Financial Interests in Human Subjects Research

All true universities, whether public or private, are public trusts designed to advance knowledge by safeguarding the free inquiry of impartial teachers and scholars. Their independence is essential because the university provides knowledge not only to its students, but also to the public agency in need of expert guidance and the general society in need of greater knowledge; and . . . these latter clients have a stake in disinterested professional opinion, stated without fear or favor, which the institution is morally required to respect.

American Association of University Professors, Declaration of principles (1915)*.

* 1 Bull. Am. Assoc. Univ. Professors 40 (Spring 1954).
Task Force on Financial Conflicts of Interest in Clinical Research
December 2001

AAMC Task Force on Financial Conflicts of Interest In Clinical Research

TASK FORCE CHAIR
William Danforth, M.D.
Chancellor Emeritus and
Vice-Chairman, Board of Trustees,
Washington University at
St. Louis
John Thomas Bigger, M.D.
Professor of Medicine and
Pharmacology, Columbia
University
Frank Davidoff, M.D.
Editor, *Annals of Internal Medicine*
Martin J. Delaney
Founding Director, Project Inform

Susan Dentzer
NewsHour with Jim Lehrer

Susan H. Ehringhaus, Esq.
Vice Chancellor and General
Counsel, University of
North Carolina at Chapel Hill

Ginger Graham
Group Chairman, Guidant
Corporation

Susan Hellmann, M.D., M.P.H.
Chief Medical Officer, Genentech

Jeffrey Kahn, Ph.D., M.P.H.
Director, Center for Bioethics,
University of Minnesota

Marvin Kalb
Executive Director, Washington
Office, Joan Shorenstein Center for
the Press, Politics and Public
Policy, John F. Kennedy School of
Government

Russel E. Kaufman, M.D.
Vice Dean, Education and
Academic Affairs, Duke University
School of Medicine

Robert P. Kelch, M.D.
Dean, University of Iowa College
of Medicine

Mark R. Laret
Chief Executive Officer, University
of California, San Francisco
Medical Center

Joan S. Leonard, Esq.

Vice President and General
Counsel, Howard Hughes Medical
Institute

Ronald Levy, M.D.
Robert K. and Helen K. Summy
Professor in the School of
Medicine, Stanford University

Constance E. Lieber
President, NARSAD

Joseph B. Martin, M.D., Ph.D.
Dean, Faculty of Medicine,
Harvard Medical School

Edward D. Miller, M.D.
Dean, Johns Hopkins School of
Medicine; CEO, Johns Hopkins
Medicine

Thomas H. Murray, Ph.D.
President and Chief Executive
Officer, The Hastings Center

Charles P. O'Brien, M.D., Ph.D.
Chief of Psychiatry, Philadelphia
Veterans Affairs Medical Center;
Kenneth Appel Professor and
Vice-Chair of Psychiatry,
University of Pennsylvania

Hon. John E. Porter, Esq.
Partner
Hogan and Hartson, L.L.P.

Roger Porter, M.D.
Vice President, Clinical Research
and Development, Wyeth-Ayerst
Research

Paul G. Ramsey, M.D.
Vice President for Medical Affairs
and Dean of the School of
Medicine, University of
Washington

Dorothy K. Robinson, Esq.
Vice President and General
Counsel, Yale University

Frances M. Visco, Esq.
President, The National Breast
Cancer Coalition

Savio Woo, Ph.D.
Director and Professor,
Institute for Gene Therapy,
Mount Sinai School of Medicine

Alastair J.J. Wood, M.D.
Assistant Vice Chancellor for
Research, Professor of Medicine,
Professor of Pharmacology,
Vanderbilt University School of
Medicine
AAU Liaison

Richard J. Turman
Director of Federal Relations,
The Association of American
Universities AAMC Staff

David Korn, M.D.
Senior Vice President, Association
of American Medical Colleges
Division of Biomedical and Health
Sciences Research

Jennifer Kulynych, J.D., Ph.D.
Director and Regulatory Counsel,
Association of American Medical
Colleges Division of Biomedical
and Health Sciences Research

The work of the Task Force was
supported in part by a grant from
the Howard Hughes Medical
Institute.

Introduction: New Recommendations to Address an Emerging Concern

Academic institutions are privileged to serve as a public trust for the advancement, preservation, and dissemination of knowledge. These institutions have diverse obligations: to students, faculty, and staff; to legislators and regulators; to donors and benefactors; and to society at large. When meeting these obligations in the ordinary course of business, institutions must and do reconcile competing interests.[21] In so doing, institutions recognize widely that policies must be made

---

[21] For example, an institution may adopt policies that require board members to disclose any financial or other personal interests in companies that transact business with the institution.

and decisions taken in a manner that is free of the taint of improper bias or conflict of interest.

Increasingly, academic institutions that conduct research also invest in – and accept the philanthropy of – commercial research sponsors. Regulators, legislators, journalists, and patient advocates have now begun to question whether such financial relationships may give rise to "institutional" conflicts of interest that could threaten research integrity and, especially troubling, potentially pose risks to human research subjects. Concern has arisen that existing institutional processes for resolving competing interests may be insufficient when the institution has a financial interest in the outcome of research and the safety and welfare of human subjects are at stake.

Although perceived risks to human subjects have received the greatest attention thus far, the growing perception that research institutions may have financial conflicts of interest also threatens to weaken public support for research. In an era of tremendous public investment in academic research, legislators and policymakers and others justifiably expect heightened public accountability from research institutions.

In a 2001 report to Congress, the General Accounting Office addressed concerns about institutional financial interests in research, noting that equity ownership or other investment in a research sponsor "may color [an institution's] review, approval, or monitoring of research conducted under its auspices or its allocation of equipment, facilities, and staff for research."[22] The GAO called upon the U.S. Department of Health and Human Services to promulgate new regulations or to issue guidance to address institutional conflicts of interest.

The AAMC's Task Force on Financial Conflicts of Interest in Clinical Research believes that an institution holding certain financial

---

[22] U.S. General Accounting Office, Biomedical Research: HHS Direction Needed to Address Financial Conflicts of Interest (GAO-02-89) (November 2001) at 7 [hereafter "GAO Report"].

interests related to its human subjects research[23] may face a conflict of interest when that institution employs the individuals who review, supervise, and conduct the research. This is especially troubling because the regulation of federally sponsored university research is centered on the principles of institutional integrity in the conduct of that research and responsibility and accountability for its oversight. Because the safety and welfare of research subjects and the objectivity of the research could be – or could appear to be – compromised whenever an institution holds a significant financial interest that could be affected by the outcome, the Task Force offers the principles and the recommended processes described in this report as a means to address an institution's competing fiduciary responsibilities and ethical obligations in the context of human subjects research.

As an initial response to a problem of remarkable complexity, this report does not provide an exhaustive list of potentially troubling financial interests; nor does it prescribe a comprehensive scheme for the oversight of all institutional relationships with commercial research sponsors. Instead, the report offers a conceptual framework for assessing institutional conflicts of interest and a set of specific recommendations for the oversight of certain financial interests in human subjects research that, in the view of the AAMC's Task Force, are especially problematic and must therefore receive close scrutiny.

The Task Force recognizes that the Association of American Universities, in its role as the representative of the leaders of major research universities, has issued recommendations on institutional conflicts of interest and continues to develop policies applicable to an

---

[23] "Human subjects research" includes all research meeting the definition of "research" performed with "human subjects" as these terms are defined in federal regulations at 45 C.F.R. Part 46 and 21 C.F.R. Part 56, without regard to the source of the research funding or whether the research is otherwise subject to federal regulation. In the event that the federal definitions of "human subject" or "research" are modified through rulemaking, any such revisions shall apply for the purpose of this guidance.

institution's financial interests in research of any type. The AAMC's Task Force believes that its own recommendations, which apply specifically to financial interests in human subjects research, complement and further develop the general recommendations issued by the AAU in its 2001 Report on Individual and Institutional Financial Conflict of Interest.[24]

I. A Framework for Assessing Institutional Conflicts of Interest in Human Subjects Research

An institution may have a conflict of interest in human subjects research whenever the financial interests of the institution, or of an institutional official acting within his or her authority on behalf of the institution, might affect – or reasonably appear to affect – institutional processes for the conduct, review, or oversight of human subjects research.

An institution conducting human subjects research may face a conflict among multiple duties or interests. Among these are a duty to protect human subjects, a duty to ensure the integrity of research and its compliance with applicable law and regulation, and the institution's legitimate interest in its own financial health and the economic viability of its academic and research missions. Institutional policies should affirm that the welfare of human subjects and the integrity of research will not be compromised – or appear to be compromised – by competing institutional interests or obligations.

Such compromise is possible when an institution fails to separate fully and reliably the responsibility for the administrative oversight of human subjects research from the responsibility for the

---

[24] Association of American Universities, Task Force on Research Accountability, Report on Individual and Institutional Financial Conflict of Interest (Oct. 2001). Among the AAU's recommendations were the following: that institutions segregate decision-making about financial and research activities so they are separately and independently managed, and that institutions establish a review group to evaluate possible conflicts arising from the financial interests of the institution and its officials.

management of certain financial interests. Institutions should ensure that the responsibility for human subjects research does not overlap or coincide with the responsibility for those institutional financial interests that may be directly affected by the outcome of the research. Individuals with authority for the immediate oversight of human subjects research, such as deans, chairs, department and laboratory heads, and IRB chairs, should not have responsibility for the management of an institution's investments or technology transfer program.[25]

As a fundamental principle, institutions should ensure that in practice, the functions and administrative responsibilities related to human subjects research are separate from those related to investment management and technology licensing.

The GAO noted in its 2001 report on financial conflicts of interest that several of the five major research institutions that it examined did attempt to separate financial and research functions, either by segregating technology transfer offices organizationally from the administration of research or by erecting "firewalls" between the management of institutional investments and academic affairs.[26] The AAMC's Task Force believes that institutions may achieve credible separation of function when technology transfer is segregated from human subjects research administration and when institutional financial interests, such as the endowment and other investments, are managed externally, through legally separate organizations.[27] When

---

[25] The Task Force recognizes that at some level of senior institutional administration – whether the office of president, vice president, or provost – responsibilities for oversight of these functions will necessarily converge.

[26] GAO Report, supra note 2, at 4.

[27] With regard to institutional investments, the Task Force distinguishes between the functions of oversight and management, and uses the term "management" to refer to day-to-day decisions about investing in individual securities, funds, etc. The Task Force recognizes that the institution's board or other governing body will typically oversee the selection of investment managers and the evaluation of manager performance.

such financial interests are managed within the institution, separation of function is more challenging and requires policies and procedures for ensuring the strict segregation of all human subjects research and investment management responsibilities.[28] Ultimately, however, each institution must determine how best to segregate human subjects research and investment management functions fully and reliably within the context of its own organization and governance structure. Implicit in the principle of separation of function is an acknowledgement that in general, circumstances in which investment and research responsibilities are formally and effectively separate do not foster institutional conflict of interest. Importantly, however, circumstances exist in which separation of function is not sufficient to avoid the appearance of institutional conflict of interest. As described in Section III, even when separation of function has been achieved, certain financial relationships with commercial sponsors should be examined closely for the presence of institutional conflict of interest. Institutions should, as a matter of prudence, establish mechanisms for formally reviewing such financial relationships and assessing the nature and extent of any conflict of interest. Moreover, where such relationships exist, institutions should presume that absent compelling circumstances and careful management of the conflict, the human subjects research in question should not be conducted at, or under the auspices of, the conflicted institution.

II. Institutional Officials

At times the institution's officers and administrators may face a conflict between a primary and professional duty – serving the

---

[28] Moses and Martin (2001) have suggested that institutions create a separate entity to hold and manage individual and institutional equity interests in research sponsors. The investment company would be overseen by a board with "wide representation," including representatives from outside the university. Hamilton Moses and Joseph B. Martin, Academic Relationships With Industry: A New Model for Biomedical Research, 2001 JAMA 285, 933.

institution – and a secondary, personal interest, namely, the possibility of individual financial gain. Personal financial interests are ordinarily governed by an institution's policies on individual conflicts of interest.

In some cases, however, an official's position may convey an authority that is so pervasive or a responsibility for research programs or administration that is so direct[29] that a conflict between the individual's financial interests and the institution's human subjects research should also be considered an "institutional conflict of interest."

Such an individual might be, for example, the dean of research, but might also be the head of a laboratory or institute or the director of a division or department in which the research is conducted, depending upon the organizational structure of the institution and the autonomy of investigators within the administrative unit.

Consequently, when an individual has the authority to make decisions that affect or reasonably appear to affect the conduct, review, or oversight of human subjects research at the institution,[30] while at the same time holding a significant financial interest in the investigational product or the research sponsor (with reference to the valuation thresholds in the 2001 AAMC guidelines on individual financial interests) an institutional conflict of interest may exist. In such cases,

---

[29] An institutional official with direct responsibility for research has the capacity, by virtue of his or her position, to reasonably affect or appear to affect the conduct, review, or oversight of current or proposed research at the institution.

[30] For example, the official may have the authority to make supervisory decisions about the institution's or administrative unit's research program, or promotion and tenure decisions regarding research faculty. Institutions may also wish to consider how best to dissuade senior faculty with significant financial interests in research sponsors from transferring pro forma responsibility for a research protocol to a junior colleague, in an attempt to avoid disclosure and oversight of financial conflicts of interest.

the individual should disclose all relevant circumstances to a superior, and if any conflicts of interest cannot be eliminated through recusal, or managed effectively via a strategy approved by the appropriate institutional committee, the research should not be conducted within or under the auspices of the institution.[31]

Beyond compliance with policies and procedures, institutional officials must foster what has been described as a "culture of conscience" in the research enterprise.[32] Exercising their authority within the institution, officials should insist upon rigorous enforcement of conflict of interest policies. Leading by personal example, officers and administrators should demonstrate to the academic community and to the public that compliance with these policies, including full disclosure of financial conflicts of interest, is an imperative reflecting core institutional values.

III. Circumstances That Ipso Facto May Create – or Appear to Create – Institutional Conflict of Interest (ICOI) in Human Subjects Research and Must Therefore Receive Close Scrutiny

It is the view of the Task Force that certain financial relationships between institutions and commercial sponsors of human subjects research may present – or appear to present – a conflict of interest, even though an institution has fully separated all of its research and investment functions. Such circumstances warrant the highest degree of scrutiny in every instance in which they occur.

---

[31]   The Task Force recognizes that some institutions have established policies governing potential conflicts of interest arising from the personal financial interests of institutional officials. If an official lacks the authority to make decisions that will affect or appear to affect the conduct, review, or oversight of research, that official's financial interests should be evaluated and, if necessary, managed or eliminated as required by an institution's applicable policies on individual conflict of interest.

[32]   Charles Marwick, New Head of Federal Office Clear on Protecting Human Research Participants, 2002 JAMA 284, 1501, 1502.

Accordingly, when one or more of the following circumstances exist, the institution should conduct a specific, fact-driven inquiry into whether the particular financial relationship may affect or reasonably appear to affect human subjects research conducted at or under the auspices of the institution:

A. When the institution is entitled to receive royalties from the sale of the investigational product that is the subject of the research;

B. When, through its technology licensing activities or investments related to such activities, the institution has obtained an equity interest or an entitlement to equity of any value (including options or warrants) in a *non-publicly traded* sponsor of human subjects research at the institution;

C. When, through technology licensing activities or investments related to such activities, the institution has obtained an ownership interest or an entitlement to equity (including options or warrants) of greater than $100,000 in value (when valued in reference to current public prices, or, where applicable, using accepted valuation methods), in a *publicly-traded* sponsor of human subjects research at the institution;[33] [see fn] or

D. When, with regard to a specific research project to be conducted at or under the auspices of the institution, institutional officials with direct responsibility for human subjects research (see Section II) hold a significant financial interest in the commercial research sponsor or the investigational product. "Significant financial interest" is defined for this purpose as one or more of the following:

   1. An equity interest or entitlement to equity (including options or warrants) of any amount in a *non-publicly traded* sponsor of

---

[33] The AAMC should periodically reassess this threshold to determine whether the amount remains appropriate for the purpose of identifying possible ICOI. The Task Force notes also that ownership interests in subsidiary companies acting as sponsors of institutional research involving human subjects may warrant scrutiny at lower threshold amounts.

human subjects research conducted at or under the auspices of the institution;

2. An equity interest or entitlement to equity (including options or warrants) in excess of the *de minimis* amount (and not including exceptions for certain mutual funds), as defined in the AAMC's 2001 guidelines for individual financial interests, in a publicly traded sponsor of human subjects research conducted at or under the auspices of the institution;

3. Consulting fees, honoraria, gifts or other emoluments, or "in kind" compensation from a sponsor of human subjects research conducted at or under the auspices of the institution, that in the aggregate exceeded the de minimis amount as defined in the AAMC's 2001 guidelines for individual financial interests, or are expected to exceed that amount in the next twelve months;

4. An appointment to serve, in either a personal or representative capacity, as an officer, director, or board member of a commercial sponsor of human subjects research conducted at or under the auspices of the institution, whether or not remuneration is received for such service; or

5. An appointment to serve on the scientific advisory board of a commercial sponsor of human subjects research conducted at or under the auspices of the institution, unless the official has no current significant financial interest in the sponsor or the investigational product and agrees not to hold such an interest for a period of no less than three years following completion of any related research conducted at or under the auspices of the institution.

IV. Other Financial Relationships That May Warrant Close Scrutiny

In addition to those circumstances identified in Section III, which must always be examined for the presence of conflict of interest, the Task Force recognizes that other financial relationships with research sponsors may warrant internal or external scrutiny, depending upon the relevant circumstances. Examples of the relationships that may fall in this category are listed below.

This list of other financial relationships that may warrant scrutiny is not intended to be exhaustive; nor does the Task Force attempt to recommend specific mechanisms for oversight of the relationships described. As a general rule, institutions should determine the nature and degree of scrutiny required for any of these relationships or interests by assessing the potential for conflict of interest and weighing the magnitude of any risk to human subjects.

The Task Force recommends that when developing policies and procedures to address potential conflicts of interest, institutions pay particular attention to the following circumstances:

A. When an investigator, research administrator, or institutional official with research oversight authority participates materially in a procurement or purchasing decision involving major purchases from, or non-routine supply contracts with, a commercial entity that sponsors human subjects research at the institution; or

B. When the institution has received substantial gifts (including gifts in kind) from a potential commercial sponsor of human subjects research. Evaluation of the potential sponsor's gift history might include the following:

☐ (1) Whether a gift is of sufficient magnitude that even when held in the general endowment for the benefit of the entire institution, it might affect, or reasonably appear to affect, oversight of human subjects research at the institution;

☐ (2) Whether a gift is held for the express benefit of the college, school, department, institute or other unit where the human subjects research is to be conducted; or

☐ (3) Whether any institutional officer who has the authority, by virtue of his or her position, to affect or appear to affect the conduct, review or oversight of the proposed human subjects research has been involved in solicitation of the gift.

Although the listed circumstances are potential areas of concern, the Task Force does not intend to preclude institutions from accepting the philanthropy of corporations that sponsor human sub-jects research. Rather, the Task Force is recommending that institu-tions develop means of identifying such circumstances and managing, through disclosure and as otherwise appropriate, any actual or appar-ent conflicts of interest that may result. In addition, the Task Force recommends that institutions adopt clear policies governing the han-dling of gifts. All gifts should be accepted in conformance with those policies and reported to the development office for record-keeping purposes. Faculty should be held accountable for adhering to gift policies.

V. Structure of ICOI Reporting and Review Process

A. Institutional Conflict of Interest (ICOI) Committee

The Task Force recommends that an institution form a standing ICOI committee for the purpose of reviewing the circumstances described in Section III (except when any conflicts of interest atten-dant to these circumstances have been resolved through recusal or oth-erwise eliminated). The Task Force recommends that the ICOI com-mittee members be individuals who have sufficient seniority, exper-tise, and independence to evaluate the competing interests at stake and make credible and effective recommendations. All members of the ICOI committee should be independent of the direct line of authority for human subjects research oversight within the institution. One or more external ("public") members are strongly urged, as the inclu-sion of public members will increase the transparency of the commit-tee's deliberations and enhance the credibility of its determinations. Recusal should be required whenever any member has an actual or apparent conflict of interest with regard to any matter under review.

Thus, an ICOI committee might include one or more members of the board of trustees, one or more individuals with no professional, personal, or financial ties to the institution, and one or more senior faculty. An ICOI committee should include one or more alternates to sit in place of any member who has recused himself or herself from the deliberations.

The Task Force recognizes that many institutions have created committees to review individual conflict of interest. Some institutions may prefer to rely upon those committees for ICOI review rather than forming separate ICOI committees. Each institution must determine which committee structure is most appropriate to its organizational structure and governance; however, the Task Force urges institutions to consider the advantages of separate committees, in view of the complexity and sensitivity of the issues to be considered by the ICOI committee, the need for participation by senior officials, and the strong recommendation that public members be included.

B. Reporting of Institutional Financial Interests Obtained Through Licensing Agreements

The institution's office of technology licensing should report to the ICOI committee (or an appropriate institutional official charged with identifying circumstances for ICOI review) when, as the result of a licensing agreement, the institution takes (or intends to take) an equity interest, stock options, or any entitlement to an owner-ship interest in, or royalty payments from, a potential sponsor of human subjects research conducted at or under the auspices of the institution.[34]

C. Reporting and Review of Personal Financial Interests of Institutional Officials

Institutional officers, board members, and administrators who over-see human subjects research – including the president, vice president for research, deans, chairs, institute heads, and the chairs of the IRB and COI committees – should be required, under institutional

---

[34] The question of whether an institution should take an equity position in a research company is a matter for the institution to decide. Institutions should, however, develop clear policies to guide such decisions, and should consider whether equity positions might create the appearance of unacceptable conflict of interest if related human subjects research were to be conducted at the institution.

policies for individual conflicts of interest, to make an annual report of any personal financial interests that might appear to be affected by human subjects research conducted at or under the auspices of the institution. (As a guide to determining *de minimis* exemptions to this policy, institutions should apply the valuation thresholds in the AAMC's 2001 guidelines for the oversight of individual financial interests in human subjects research.)

The financial reports of institutional officials with research oversight responsibilities should be received by the institution's COI or ICOI committees (or their designated representatives), as appropriate, or, in the case of senior officers and board members, by the audit or other committee or subcommittee of the board, or its designee. The reviewing committee should determine whether significant financial interests in an investigational product or in a sponsor of human subjects research may be managed effectively or should be eliminated. All such decisions should be documented and communicated to the individual and his or her superior. When the COI or ICOI committee determines that an official should be permitted to hold a significant financial interest in an investigational product or commercial research sponsor even though the official will not be formally recused from research-related responsibilities, this information should be communicated to the IRB of record.

D. Rebuttable Presumption Against Certain Institutional Financial Interests in Human Subjects Research

When reviewing any of the circumstances described in Section III, the ICOI committee should apply a rebuttable presumption against conduct of the human subjects research at or under the auspices of the institution. The presumption may be rebutted when the circumstances are compelling and the committee has approved an effective conflict management plan. Whether the ICOI committee deems the circumstances to be compelling should depend in each case upon the nature of the science, the nature of the interest, how closely the interest is related to the research, the degree of risk that the research poses to human subjects, and the degree to which the interest may be affected by the research. The committee should consider whether the institution is uniquely qualified, by virtue of its attributes (e.g., special facilities or equipment, unique patient population) and the experience and expertise of its investigators, to conduct the research and safeguard the welfare of the human subjects involved.

Even when the institution is deemed uniquely qualified, conflicts associated with significant risk to human subjects should be avoided whenever possible and, if permitted, should be managed closely.

E. Report of Institutional Conflicts of Interest to the Institutional Review Board

After reviewing a significant financial interest in research, the ICOI committee should communicate its conclusions, along with any management conditions to be imposed, to the institutional review board(s) having jurisdiction over the research. All relevant conflicts should be disclosed to research subjects in a form to be determined by the IRB of record.

VI. Additional Recommendations

A. *Multi-center Trials.* When the institution holds one of the financial interests described in Section III and any conflicts of interest will not be eliminated through recusal or otherwise, the presumption should be that the institution will not conduct related human subjects research except as the non-primary site in a multi-center trial. Even when participating as other than the primary site in a multi-center trial, the institution should not serve as the coordinating site unless the possible institutional conflicts of interest described in Section III have been eliminated.

B. *External Monitoring of Single/Primary Site Trials.* Serving as the sole or primary performance site might be justified under compelling circumstances (e.g., when the research is an early-stage or feasibility trial *and* the expertise of institutional investigators is essential to the research). In such a case, however, the ICOI committee should approve the circumstances, and if advisable, the research should be subject to monitoring by an oversight body with external members (e.g., a data and safety monitoring board).

C. *External IRB Review*. When the ICOI committee has determined that compelling circumstances exist as described in Section V.D (above), the institution should consider the desirability of contracting with an external IRB to provide a second level of review and oversight.

D. *Recusal*. The committee that reviews financial reports of institutional officials should have the authority to recommend that formal recusal be required when an official holds a significant financial interest in an investigational product or in an entity sponsoring human subjects research. The scope of this recusal should include any involvement in matters or decisions that might reasonably appear to affect the research. Recusal is not an effective management strategy when the individual, by virtue of conflicts arising from personal financial holdings, would be precluded from fulfilling the responsibilities of his or her position. In such cases, the best interests of the institution may necessitate that the individual divest the interests or vacate the position.

E. *Interim Recusal*. If an institutional official who holds a significant financial interest in an investigational product or commercial research sponsor becomes aware that he or she must take an action or participate in a decision that may affect or reasonably appear to affect the institution's human subjects research, and the official has not yet been directed by the ICOI committee (or COI committee, if applicable) to recuse himself or herself from the matter, the official should be required to disclose the circumstances to his or her superior. The superior may determine that recusal is necessary, may decline to require recusal, or may refer the matter to the ICOI committee for resolution. When the superior declines to require recusal, the reviewing committee should make the final determination as to whether recusal is in fact necessary. In any case, the superior should document his or her recusal determination and forward this documentation to the ICOI committee. The ICOI should maintain a central repository of information about all recusal determinations related to the institution's human subjects research.

F. *Hospital as a Separate Entity.* At times the institution's faculty, staff, or students may conduct human subjects research at affiliated, yet legally separate, hospitals or clinical sites. The Task Force recommends that all affiliates operating under the institution's Federal-Wide Assurance (FWA) for the protection of human subjects agree to abide by ICOI policies that are the same as or no less stringent than those adopted by the institution.

G. *Accreditation.* The effectiveness of an institution's ICOI policies and a formal assessment of the institution's compliance with these policies should be examined as an element of any accreditation process for the institution's human subjects protection program.

VII. IRB Members

A. Applying the threshold valuation levels in the AAMC's 2001 guidelines for the oversight of individual financial interests, the institution should require that IRB members report annually any personal and significant financial interests that might reasonably appear to be affected by the scope of their responsibilities. These reports should include significant financial interests in sponsors of human subjects research when the IRB member is aware that the company in question is or may become a sponsor of human subjects research at the institution. The reports of IRB members should be reviewed by the institution's COI committee (i.e., the committee charged with reviewing the financial interests of faculty investigators), which should apply a presumption against significant individual financial interests in an investigational product or a commercial sponsor of the institution's human subjects research,[35] and stipulate that the member should

---

[35]   As described in the *2001 Guidelines*.

recuse himself or herself in any such circumstance, as described in VII.B.

B. IRB members are required by federal regulation to recuse themselves from voting upon or participating in any deliberations concerning protocols in which they have conflicting interests. Institutional policies should reiterate that disclosure and recusal are required on a protocol-by-protocol basis for all IRB members. Institutions should require the IRB administrator to poll the IRB about potentially conflicting financial interests prior to the start of each meeting and to document members' responses in the meeting minutes. Institutions should consider providing the IRB administrator with a list of the research sponsors in which one or more IRB members hold a significant financial interest, to ensure that recusal occurs when necessary.

VIII. Disclosure

Disclosure to the IRB of record, to research subjects, and in all publications should be required whenever the institution holds a financial interest (as described in Section III) that is or could reasonably appear to be in conflict with a proposed human subjects research project under the terms of these policy recommendations, and the conflict has not been eliminated through recusal or otherwise.

The IRB of record should specify the form and content of the disclosure. When the financial interests of institutional officials are or could reasonably appear to be in conflict with the institution's human subjects research, disclosure should be required unless the official has been formally recused from participation in all matters that may affect or reasonably appear to affect the conduct, review, or oversight of the research.

Conclusion

The principles and processes articulated in this document should assist institutions in their oversight of financial interests that could have, or reasonably be perceived to have, an inappropriate effect upon human subjects research. The policy recommendations offered here are more expansive than current legal requirements or standard institutional practices. With the publication of this report, the Task Force aspires to assist the academic community in responding voluntarily and credibly to the emerging concern over institutional conflicts of interest in human subjects research. In tandem with the AAMC's *2001 Policy and Guidelines for the Oversight of Individual Financial Interest in Human Subjects Research*, these new *2002 Principles and Recommendations for the Oversight of an Institution's Financial Interests in Human Subjects Research* will contribute to maintaining public trust in the research enterprise and retaining the confidence of those who generously volunteer to participate in research.

Appendix II
Glossary

ACCME	Accreditation Council for Continuing Medical Education
ACGME	Accreditation Council for Graduate Medical Education
AMA	American Medical Association
AMC	academic medical center
CMA	Canadian Medical Association
CME	continuing medical education
CRO	contract research organization
DDMAC	Division of Drug Marketing, Advertising and Communications
DTCA	direct-to-consumer advertising
FDA	Food and Drug Administration
IRB	Institutional Review Board
MECC	medical education communication companies
PCR	pharmaceutical company representative
PDR	*Physicians' Desk Reference*
PhRMA	Pharmaceutical Research and Manufacturers of America
PI	pharmaceutical industry
PPIIs	physician–pharmaceutical industry interactions
SMO	site management organization

Index

Printed in the United States
By Bookmasters